WITHDRAWN

W9-BDT-159

# My Spirit Took You In

# My Spirit Took You In

### The Romance that Sparked an Epidemic of Fear

## LOUISE TROH

WITH CHRISTINE WICKER

ELISHA D. SMITH PUBLIC LIBRARY
MENASHA, WISCONSIN

WEINSTEIN
BOOKS

Copyright © 2015 by Louise Troh

All rights reserved. No part of this book may be used or reproduced in
any manner whatsoever without the written permission of the Publisher.
For information address Weinstein Books, 250 West 57th Street,
15th Floor, New York, NY 10107.

Printed in the United States of America.

Library of Congress Cataloging-in-Publication Data is available for this book.

Editorial production by *Marra*thon Production Services.
www.marrathon.net

· BOOK DESIGN BY JANE RAESE
Set in 12-point New Baskerville

ISBN 978-1-60286-289-0 (print)
ISBN 978-1-60286-290-6 (e-book)

Published by Weinstein Books
A member of the Perseus Books Group
www.weinsteinbooks.com

Weinstein Books are available at special discounts for bulk purchases
in the U.S. by corporations, institutions and other organizations.
For more information, please contact the Special Markets Department
at the Perseus Books Group, 2300 Chestnut Street, Suite 200,
Philadelphia, PA 19103, call (800) 810-4145, ext. 5000,
or e-mail special.markets@perseusbooks.com.

FIRST EDITION

10 9 8 7 6 5 4 3 2 1

TO AMERICA, AFRICA, AND THE WORLD

# CONTENTS

# CHAPTER ONE

# A Man Completely

I stayed in a chair as Eric Duncan crossed my living room in Dallas, Texas. It was about 10:00 p.m. on September 20, 2014. I had not seen him in sixteen years.

He was over six feet tall, with a shaved head. I am not such a big woman, five feet and four inches. I stood up and greeted him. "You are so big."

This was not such a good thing to say for my first sentence, but it was all I thought of. He was so skinny when we met twenty years ago. At that time, Thomas Eric Duncan, known to everyone as Eric, was barely a man. Exiles on the run from the war in our country, Liberia, we lived with thousands of others in a refugee encampment in Danané, a city in the Ivory Coast. Then Eric was a kind almost-man growing into a gentle grown man.

Eric was one of many people I loved in my life, but always I loved him special. I can't say why; it was like God picked us for each other. Our spirits knew each other from that first day when he called out to me on a dusty road in Danané.

In my living room Eric said, "I thought you would be bigger, eating all this American food."

"You can't eat everything here or you will be too big," I told him.

We were nervous.

Eric's face was broader now. He was older but the same. He had some gray in his beard, but when I looked at him I could see both men: the young one from the Ivory Coast and this older one, tired from his travels, who had wanted us to be together for so long.

When Eric came to Dallas I was afraid he would not love me when he saw how old I'd become. I was fifty-four years old, ten years more than him. My legs hurt. Gray was coming into my hair. I worked as a certified nurse assistant at a senior living center. My hands were rough from so much Clorox, so many years of cleaning. Dishes. Pots. Sinks. Diapers. Toilets. Floors. Cleaning everything. And the next day, cleaning again.

Over the years I told Eric many times that I was too old for him; but he said no, never. And I had laughed, the soft African laugh that has only a little sound and means all is well. It means we are together in this thinking, but I am waiting to see what will happen. Laughing sometimes tells more than words.

I told him that I needed to protect my heart. It was old and tired, and I could not risk it again.

On the phone he said, "I will not hurt you. I will make you happy. Let me try."

Afraid to hope, I said nothing.

Since the days we'd met in the Ivory Coast he had loved me. Always he said, "You are my wife. It doesn't matter where you are. You are the mother of my son, the love of my life."

In the Ivory Coast I was a woman who had to be tough, because I was a mother with children to feed. I was skinny then, legs like sticks, dried-out skin, refugee-ugly. I could not be gentle with the world. A mother must be a tiger so that her children can survive. A mother who has nothing to give her children must give them her whole spirit. She must never let anything scare her so much that she will not defend those she loves.

I learned these things from war and exile, and then from living in America, where life is good but not as easy as Liberians think it is. When I came to America in 1998 as a political refugee, I left Eric, our son, Karsiah, and all eight of my other children in Africa. Nine children, Americans say with wide eyes; they can't believe it. I had ten in all; now nine are living.

There was no birth control in Africa. In high school, I'd been the smart girl, so mean to other girls when they were pregnant. I would say they should stay home and be pregnant, forget school. I wouldn't even sit with them. But young women fall in love and sometimes not with the right men. Before high school was over, I was pregnant myself. I could not continue with classes. I stopped going to school. But my father welcomed me in his home. He protected me and my baby.

In war, many fathers die or disappear. Some of my children's fathers had gone that way. Eric was still with me, a refugee in the Ivory Coast, when word came in 1998 that I could come to America. But I could not take him or my children with me. The visa was for one person only, not for a family. Alone is the only way. We leave our husbands and our wives, we leave our children, because only by leaving can we give them any hope for a better life.

Many years I worked to bring my children from Africa to America. I'd brought the youngest, Eric's son, Karsiah, in 2006 when he was ten. In 2005 and 2006, I'd brought four of Karsiah's older sisters. Only one sister, Kebeh Jallah, was left in Liberia. But she died before the visa came. No visa: such hopeless words. Three sons remained behind. I hoped I would see them again someday. My tenth child, Timothy, was born in America.

The big dreams of Eric's life were coming to America and being with me. In all the years apart, neither of us ever matched that love from long ago with anyone else. It would not die. I gave up on ever having him in my life, but he never gave up on us.

Sometimes over the years Eric's mother called to say that I must send her son money. She is in North Carolina now. Why did she not call her other children? Always, it seems she called me. From the first time so many years ago when she saw me dancing down the street with other people—all of us dancing and playing music, going house to house the way Africans do sometimes—not being such a good dancer, just having fun, she saw my heart. Her son did, too. He knew my self.

When relatives and friends call me from Liberia pouring desperate words into my ears, I send them what they ask for. Sometimes it was Eric's mother who called and sometimes it was Eric himself calling me, pleading. Maybe he was ashamed, but he was needing that money so much that he could not be prideful. He had other girlfriends who'd made it to America. Some of them would have their husband answer the phone or they would not answer at all. Maybe they'd say yes, but then not send the money.

"He is so desperate," Eric's mother would say. "You can remember how it is there."

Yes, I remember: boiling leaves to eat; rubbing leaves on your skin because you have no soap; crushing leaves under your arms so that you don't smell bad. Leaves and dirt, sticks and rocks: these are the only things a refugee can count on. Even if the exiles go home, the average wage in Liberia is $1.25 a day. Many people have no clean water or flush toilets. Their lives are hard every day. There is no route to riches. To get money from America is like a blessing from God—bread falling from the sky.

The desperate ones who call me now never know how hard I work in America. I don't tell them. I always send money. If I need that money for food, I pinch back what I eat. I have felt what these people are feeling.

Now Eric was finally here, was in Texas, bigger and so real—a man completely. In my living room he looked into my eyes—so closely he looked. And I saw him then again: I saw his good heart, still the same, there in his eyes, waiting for me to claim it.

He hugged me. When I sat down he sat next to me, put his arms around me, and pulled me close to him. It felt so strange to be with him at last. I knew him from so much talking on the phone, and the sharing of so many dreams. I hid Eric's love at the center of my life for many years. For so many years, he was only a voice talking from so far away, many times talking about how fine our son was becoming.

Our son, Karsiah, is named for his African grandfather; he was our pride. He was the reason Eric was coming to America now. Karsiah, this boy who had not seen his father in sixteen years, was the one who finally asked Eric to come to me.

We started to think about bringing Eric here from Liberia in the fall of 2013 when Karsiah was a senior in a Dallas high school. Eric had called to talk to Karsiah so many times over the years, sometimes every day. Our son felt his love and wanted him at his graduation. The principal of Karsi-ah's school wrote a letter to the American Embassy telling of Karsiah's graduation and supporting the visa application. The principal's efforts paid off. The visa was granted, but it came through on July 25, 2014, too late for the graduation.

Eric always worked hard, but Liberians don't make enough money to pay for plane tickets; I would pay for it. However, by the time Eric's visa came through in July, the money I had for his May ticket was gone. Eric's half sister had agreed to pay for his ticket, but in August she admitted that she wasn't going to. I didn't have enough money, but a person in the Liberian community will loan people money for such things. I borrowed $2,000 for Eric's ticket.

I would pay off the debt plus $500 from my tax returns. Eric's nephew Oliver gave me $400 from his paycheck to help purchase the ticket. First I tried to get a ticket for a flight in early September, but it was taken. The next ticket was for September 19; I bought it. When Eric got the ticket, he was so happy. Our talks then started to be not about what we had done or even what we were doing, but about our plans. We were old now. But we could be together. We would make a life at last.

On his way to Dallas—and to me—Eric called from each airport where he landed on his journey. In Liberia as he was about to leave, he rang to say, "I am on my way at last, sweetheart."

He sounded so happy. And me? I was cautious.

In Brussels he called again: "I am getting closer."

I didn't go to the airport to meet Eric; I waited in the apartment. As I waited, I wondered what he would think of this new life I was bringing him to.

I lived in Vickery Meadow, a Dallas neighborhood filled with about a hundred big apartment complexes. In the 1970s, Vickery Meadow was popular for young single people with good jobs, but in the 1980s when Dallas had an oil bust and a real estate bust at the same time, wealthier people started moving to other areas. Twenty-five thousand people, mostly immigrants speaking more than twenty-seven languages, now live in about two and a half square miles, such a packed-in place that one journalist called it "an anthill." Maybe this newspaper writer also meant that we are swarming everywhere on the streets of Vickery Meadow.

That's not exactly how it is, but people from other parts of the city may think that a half dozen people walking down a block is a swarm. In most Dallas neighborhoods, nobody is outside at all. The city is so spread out, and everyone is in cars. In Vickery Meadow some people don't have money for cars, so they walk or wait in little groups for buses. Most people on the street there have dark skin, and if they speak English, it is with an accent. I thought the things that make lots of people in Dallas nervous might make Eric feel at home. Or maybe he would feel lost in all these different kinds of people.

I didn't have to tell Eric these thoughts to know what he would say: "I am coming to be with you, to love you and to love your family."

My neighbors and I were poor by Dallas standards, and some people thought of us as troublesome. Crime was bad in the 1990s, but the city set up a neighborhood improvement district so security patrols could help keep criminals away. Forty social-service agencies help people in Vickery Meadow. But my neighborhood might not look so poor to a man coming from Africa. In Liberia, Eric rented one small room in a tin-roofed house in a town outside of Monrovia, the capital. He had no car.

In Dallas I had a 2009 silver Toyota Corolla. Without a car, it would have been hard for me to travel five miles to the Windsor Senior Living Center where I was a certified nurse assistant. I learned to drive only after I came to Dallas. It still made me nervous, but I was a safe driver, never speeding, sometimes being honked at by Mexicans for not moving fast enough.

My four daughters, who live near me and bring their children to see me nearly every day, told me to speed up. But I said, "No. I am not going to have a wreck. Let these people get as mad as they want."

Eric had never been out of Africa, and he had never seen people from so many countries as he would see in Vickery Meadow. Managers at the Ivy Apartments where I live say eight languages are spoken just in my complex. But Eric might never get to know the neighbors. Not to know neighbors is the Dallas way, and that is okay. I had so many relatives coming and going, Eric would be able to make many Liberian friends. Many of Dallas's 10,000 Liberians live in Vickery Meadow. I know a lot of them and they know me. At Conrad High School, where our son, Karsiah, was a quarterback, the football team is almost all Liberian.

Vickery Meadow is in a good location, not too far from rich neighborhoods where people need yard work and cleaning service. There are lots of bus lines for people to go to work and lots of stores: Walmart, Target, JCPenney, and best of all, Fiesta Grocery. Africans, Mexicans, Indians, Chinese—everybody likes to shop at Fiesta because it has foods from the countries we left: catfish, yams, okra, hot spices, cactus leaves, mangos, so much more food than grocery stores in Africa. This grocery store is not as pretty as the more expensive ones. It feels more like where we came from.

Eric will be so amazed to see vegetables, meat, and fish all piled so high and so many aisles of food in cans and packages with languages that are not English. You get lost just looking. Eric ran a little grocery when he lived in Ghana, just cigarettes, toilet paper, and some food that he sold from his house. Almost no stores like that exist in Dallas—maybe none at all. This way of working to make a little money is not so possible in America, but Eric says he has bigger plans. He has skills and always he is talking, talking about what jobs he will have when he gets here.

Eric was a man who could do many things, educated in computers. He was a mechanic and an electrician. He loved to work, was not lazy. But most of his life was in exile. Nobody wants to hire refugees. Nobody gives them rights. When civil war in our country finally ended, he went home to Liberia from the Ivory Coast, but so much was gone. Our lovely little country was burned and bombed until almost nothing remained. Some men suffering so hard a life would be angry and bitter, but Eric always said some positive thing. No matter how hard life was, he thought of what was good.

My two-bedroom apartment was Number 614, on the second floor of the Ivy Apartments. If there was ivy growing anywhere, I had not seen it. No buildings are tall in Vickery Meadow, all low; three stories is the highest. The apartments look like giant motels sprawling over parking lots. There is a little grass, some trees, but mostly concrete with cracks and holes and grease spots, and cars crawling through them all the time. An iron fence circles most apartments. Everything is gray and brown and tan.

People in Africa believe that Americans have so much money. Eric might have expected me to have many more possessions than I did or to live in a big house with a yard like people he sees on television. The first thing he would notice in my apartment was a picture of Jesus praying in the Garden of Gethsemane the night before he was crucified. I thumbtacked it to the wall that faced the outside door so it was the first thing I saw when I came in. I didn't have other pictures on my walls like some Americans do.

In African houses that Eric was used to, everything was plain, with not much furniture, no pictures to make the walls look pretty, no lamps sitting around, just rooms where lots of people could be together.

To one side of the wall with the picture of Jesus was the kitchen. If Eric looked in my kitchen, he would see many pots and pans, all of them big. I bought the biggest ones I could find so that I could cook lots of food. The father of one of my sons, Timothy, told a reporter that I used food to lure people to my house.

I laughed at that idea. I did not cook special food for Eric before he came, but I would cook for him later. I did not dress in any special way. Maybe I was too nervous to make a fuss yet. I was mostly concerned about my son Timothy, thirteen years old. Eric is not his father.

I talked to Timothy before Eric left Liberia. "Your father and I could not get along," I told him. "So we had to part. Now Eric is coming. He will love you like you are his own son."

"Will he do things for me? Will he take me to the mall?" Timothy asked.

"Yes, he will. He will buy you many things, the shoes you like." And then Timothy smiled.

On the kitchen side of the apartment was the bedroom shared by Timothy and two young men. I call both these men my nephews or "the boys." Neither of them is actually my nephew in the way Americans understand, but African ways of looking at family are larger. One young man, Jeffrey Cole, is a nephew of my Liberian daughter's husband. He is twenty-eight and came to Dallas from Liberia on September 3, just seventeen days before Eric arrived.

The other is Oliver Smallwood, twenty-two, who is actually Eric's nephew. He had come from Ghana in maybe 2002 and was living in North Carolina with Eric's family. At that time, Eric was living alone in Liberia in the room he rented, with none of his family near. His brother Wilfred Smallwood, Oliver's father, lives in Phoenix. His sister Mai Wureh and his mother, Nowai Korkoyah, live outside Charlotte, though his father and three other siblings remain in Africa. It's a mystery why they could get visas to come to America and Eric tried for so long and couldn't. He never entered the visa lottery in Liberia for lack of a high school education, which is required. And there was the matter of paying for the plane ticket; Eric never had the money.

Eric's mother had been calling me for a long time asking me to let Eric's nephew Oliver come to live with me. Oliver knew his cousin Karsiah when they were both small children. When he left me to go to college many miles away, Karsiah had the idea that more people should be living with me.

I think Karsiah told these boys to come here because he was worried I would be too lonely with only Timothy to cook for. Maybe he was also thinking that these nephews would get jobs and help me pay my bills. Africans usually share what money they have, and we like lots of people in our houses. Our families live together several generations at a time. Nobody thinks it strange if children in their twenties and thirties live with their parents and grandparents.

I consider Oliver my nephew, just as Eric considers my children from other fathers as his children. Although Eric and I were never married under civil law, people in Africa considered us husband and wife under customary law. To the African way of thinking, when two people have a son, that is a bond stronger than any mere civil marriage could ever be. We remain bonded to the fathers of our children and their families in a special way, even if we aren't together with the fathers. When we change partners we give our allegiance to the new partners, but the fathers of our children keep a special place within the extended family.

Maybe because African men can have many wives under customary law, we don't make a lot of difference about whether our siblings are from both mother and father or just one. Our sense of kinship is wide and deep. Even when someone hasn't been with a person in their family, or when a person is related only through marriage, we claim each other. If we are asked, we try to help one another.

On the other side of my place in the Ivy Apartments was a big living room with a blue carpet. My bedroom opened from one wall of the living room and was almost totally filled with a king-size bed. The living room had a tall wooden entertainment center, very nice, holding the fifty-five-inch TV that my oldest daughter, Youngor Jallah, had saved to buy me. Youngor is a certified nurse assistant like me. She has three boys and one girl. They live in Vickery Meadow, too.

Also in the living room of my apartment was a table for eating and a computer at one side. I stopped the Internet and the cable TV—too expensive. But Eric won't see that. Maybe all he will see is the big room and the big television.

I didn't have sofas anymore, just chairs—too many chairs. I had sofas until a little while ago. I have so many children in my apartment, so many grandchildren and friends of grandchildren who get sick and throw up. They bring food—ice cream and Coke and chocolate—and then spill it. I don't make people eat at the table, and children and cloth sofas don't always work.

Finally, those sofas were so dirty that I threw them out. I was planning to move to another apartment in a few weeks, so there was no need to replace them until I was in a new place.

Money is always tight. I went to Walmart and bought a few folding chairs. That made people think I wanted chairs. My daughter Nunser Jallah, who has two sons and lives within a few blocks of me, bought me some. Then Peterson Wayne, father of Timothy, saw office chairs at a yard sale and bought three of those. They had rollers on the legs, and the grandchildren loved to roll about the big room. I couldn't tell Nunser or Peterson to take their chairs back. That would be too rude, not grateful for their gifts. By the time Eric arrived, I had about twenty chairs in my living room.

And mattresses: I also had three mattresses there. I got so many mattresses in the same way I got the chairs. The children came over to spend the night, and they wanted to watch TV. I often keep Youngor's children because she works in the night when I am home. There wasn't room for the grown-ups and the children on the sofas. I didn't like children sleeping on the carpet, so I put out a mattress. Soon there were two more mattresses. They didn't look so good maybe, but people liked to lie on them. Eric might think all this strange furniture was so odd.

When his plane landed in Washington, DC, he called me again: "I am in America at last."

He was on his way to me. I thought of hiding some of the chairs and mattresses at my children's houses, but then the room would be so empty. Nowhere to sit. Nowhere for the children to lie down. Maybe Eric wouldn't be so surprised. He might remember that I was always just thinking about what people needed. When I was a girl in Liberia before the war came, I would always bring anyone who looked lost or sick home with me. If anyone in my family said that we didn't have food to feed them, I would say, "I'll just put them in my room so they can be safe."

Then maybe I would sneak some food to them, or they would feel better and leave. Sometimes their relatives came to find them and everyone was so happy.

Finally on the evening of September 20, Eric called again, this time from Dallas: "I am here. You can come to get me," he said.

He had no idea how far the airport was from where we lived in Northeast Dallas. So when my daughter Nopie Do-poe and my niece Amanda Jallah went to pick him up, they didn't arrive quickly, and he called me again to let them know where they could find him. He offered to help by driving the car back for them. In Liberia, Eric worked as a driver for the manager of a shipping company in Monrovia. He was a good driver for Liberia, but not for Dallas.

"You will need a while to get to know the traffic before you drive here," I told him.

He had seen America in movies. Africans have so many ideas about how it is to live in this land, but there is plenty more they do not know. At least Eric would not be cold at first. Dallas in September is warm, sometimes hot. I had arrived first in Boston, where it was so very cold. Eric did not know about American cold. I knew he couldn't imagine it.

Eric was sitting on the little chairs in baggage claim wearing a T-shirt, jeans, and a jacket. A black satchel hung from a strap across his chest. When he saw my daughter Nopie, he stood, opened his arms wide and came toward her, saying, as he always had, "My daughter." He remembered her from the days when we were together in Africa. I have a picture of her then, when she was three or four, thin and sad in a white cotton dress.

When she sees that picture, Nopie always thinks, "Sad and hungry." She isn't hungry anymore. Africans are right about that much. It is easier to find enough food in America. To go to the airport, Nopie wore a bright yellow dress and her hair dyed yellow to match. She looked like a queen.

Eric looked good, too—healthy. "He didn't even look like he came from Africa," Nopie said later. A lot of people said that: in those first days he was so healthy. The girls took Eric's rolling black bag, and they started the last part of his journey toward the home we would have together.

Nopie came behind Eric into my house, rolling his bag. Timothy was spending the night at my daughter's house.

He was still frowning about this new man, wondering if he would take away my attention too much.

When Eric came in, Jeffrey Cole and Eric's nephew Oliver Smallwood went forward to shake his hand, but his eyes found me and he came in my direction. After Eric sat with me a while, he leaned over to kiss me. But I pulled away. I stood up and looked at our nephews who were still in the room, now sitting quietly.

"I don't want to kiss here," I said. Taking him by the hand, I led him to the bedroom. When I shut the door, he turned to me and took me into his arms.

And he said, "Oh, sweetheart, you can never know how long I have dreamed of this moment."

When I looked into his face, for the first time in many months I felt that life might be good.

# CHAPTER TWO

# A Diamond in the Dirt

I first saw Thomas Eric Duncan one day in 1994 when I was walking to the Danané market. We were living in the Ivory Coast with hundreds of thousands of other Liberian refugees. Some people have said we were in a refugee camp, but it wasn't a camp, just a town with villages around it where thousands of Liberians had come, running from the civil war back home.

To find love in such a hard place as Danané is like finding a diamond in the dirt. You are so surprised to see it, you can't believe it's real. If you get to keep it, you feel so lucky. You carry it with you sometimes hidden, and sometimes so everyone can see it, but it is always the most shining thing you have. It might be the *only* beautiful thing you have.

Liberians ran to the Ivory Coast because of the terrible things that soldiers were doing to the people of my country. Lots of people there lost loved ones. The war began in 1989 and only really ended in 2003. By the end of it, 700,000 Liberians had left a country that had only 2 million people when the wars started. About 5 percent of all Liberians were killed in the wars. Some refugees are still in

Ghana, some are in Guinea, and some remain in the Ivory Coast.

In Danané there was a United Nations feeding station where we could get some food, maybe some rice or corn meal and *cocodolo*—corn dust and oil. No vegetables. No meat. We had to find our own places to live. If people had nothing and no place to live, they would find friends or relatives. Liberians help each other.

Before the war, I was living in Nimba County in the north-central part of the country. It is an area rich in iron ore, which made it so valuable to the government, and that was one reason there was so much fighting there. It was a lovely place, green with lots of rain, and some swamps. It is easy to grow food there. A mining company there called LAMCO, the Liberian-American-Swedish Minerals Company, was established before I was born or maybe when I was a little girl. I can't remember a time before this big company with offices and a mine and houses came to Liberia.

Everyone there was white, from different countries: Germany, France, America, and England. A lot of good things came from this company, but when the war started it shut down and all the white people went away.

People in Liberia say that the war happened because the country boys got tired of being bossed around by the city boys. By "city boys" we mean a very small part of the population, maybe 5 percent, called Americo-Liberians and sometimes Congos, and sometimes just Negroes. These people are descended from former slaves and free blacks from America who were resettled in Liberia by American reformers in the mid-1800s. These black Americans set up a capital city they named Monrovia, after President James

Monroe. They formed a republic in 1847 and quickly started ruling over the tribal Africans.

These Americans looked down on the native Africans and used them as slaves whenever they could, which was mostly when they were children. My father was one of those children raised by Congos. Instead of sending him to school, they used him for work. When he grew up, he left to have his own life.

Officially, there were two civil wars: 1989–1997 and 1999–2003. But to many of us the wars really started in 1979, in April, the steamiest month of the Liberian year, over increases in the price of rice. People rioted in Monrovia that month and government troops controlled by Americo-Liberian president William R. Tolbert fired on demonstrators, killing hundreds.

Almost exactly one year later, a master sergeant in the army and member of the Krahn tribe named Samuel Doe killed Tolbert and took over the government. For the first time, Liberia had a tribal president; but now the horrors were spreading. Ten days later, thirteen men were publicly executed before a cheering crowd of Liberians. People started being stopped by soldiers who demanded that they speak one of the sixteen Liberian tribal languages. Because most Americo-Liberians didn't know tribal languages, they could be singled out, beaten, arrested, and even killed.

After an attempted coup in 1985 by a general from the Gio tribe in Nimba County, President Doe began to repress Gio people, my family's tribe. At this time, I had a baby and I was still swollen from pregnancy. I could hardly walk. My brother knew that violence was about to come to where we lived.

He came to me and said, "We must go somewhere safer."

But my stomach was so big and sagging down that I could hardly walk at all. So my brother carried me with the baby and put me into the car so that we could run away.

In 1989, Charles Taylor, a former supporter of Samuel Doe who had left Liberia and trained as a guerrilla in Libya, came into Liberia with an army he put together in the Ivory Coast. As the fighting expanded all over the country, I was big and pregnant with another baby. This one was so big, but still wouldn't come. So I left Nimba County for the hospital in Bong County, over eight hours from where I lived. I needed to have that baby before it got any bigger.

When I heard there was fighting near where my children were, I demanded to go home to Nimba County. On the way back from the hospital, the car was stopped by soldiers with guns who were checking people's identification. I was lucky that my ID did not say Nimba County. If people were going there, the soldiers took them away and killed them.

When they asked, I said I was going to Grand Gedeh County, the county where President Doe came from. They let me go. But I was not able to get back to my children right away. So, after some days I was going to charter a car. Five boys were also trying to charter a car, and they wanted me to go with them. But it was getting so late and dark.

I said, "No. I will wait."

They chartered a car, and the next day we found their bodies right at the gate where they would be getting on the road. All five had been beheaded.

In September 1990, Charles Taylor's ally Prince Johnson, who was from Nimba County, captured President Doe and tortured and killed him. Now no one was safe. Fighting was everywhere. Soldiers killed whole villages of people who weren't doing anything wrong. Some people claimed that the soldiers ate human flesh because they thought it gave them power.

They recruited teenage boys, gave them drugs, and taught them to rape, torture, and massacre people. Some of them wore women's clothes and acted so crazy that no one knew what horrible things they might do. People told of seeing their neighbors disemboweled. Children's hands and arms were chopped off by Charles Taylor's rebels, who would ask first, "Do you want short sleeves or long sleeves?" If they said short sleeves, their forearms were cut off. If they said long sleeves, only their hands were cut off. Babies were bashed to the earth. Pregnant women had knives stuck in their bellies to kill them and their babies. It was all done to terrify the people. And it worked.

One day, soldiers cut off the ear of a young man who was a fisherman. I had bought fish from him many times. He would say, "Just pick which fish you want to buy." And when I would pick some really big fish, he would say, "One dollar. Or a dollar and half." Not much for so much fish. He was a nice man.

But the soldiers cut off his ear when he had done nothing to them at all. When they cut off a person's ear, it meant that they were going to kill him. They wouldn't kill him right away, but cutting off the ear meant a death sentence. After they cut off the fisherman's ear, they took him away. They dragged him along the ground and beat him until his whole body was covered in blood.

I was passing when I saw him there with the soldiers. When the poor man saw me, he called out, "Help me, sister. You know me. Plead for me, that they will spare my life."

So the soldiers said to me, "Do you know this man?"

He was looking at me, calling my name. I said, "Yes. I know him."

So the soldiers said, "Then it is you who must kill him."

But I would not. I told them, "I am not going to kill him. I am not a fighter. Why would I take somebody's life away? I have my kids. I have my brothers and sisters."

So they said, "Get out of here. And don't look back."

Maybe they let me go because they were short of bullets. After I left, they cut the man's throat.

Another time during the war, I told a man who was coming to my house that he and his men were doing wrong things. They were supposed to be fighting other men, but instead they were killing innocent people.

That man said I was a troublemaker with a big mouth and that I didn't need to live. The next day he ordered me to be in my house by 4:00 that afternoon so that he could come and kill me. I went to my house and waited but he didn't come. The next morning, I waited until 9:00 a.m. and then went out to dump the bucket I used as a toilet. I heard that the man had gotten into a fight with a man on his side of the war and had gotten killed. So my life was spared.

My brother, the one who carried me to the car after I had the baby, was killed by the soldiers in Monrovia. He was twenty-five years old when the soldiers told him that he must fight with them, but my brother was a Jehovah's Witness, very religious. The Witnesses are strict and do not believe in fighting. When my brother would not join the soldiers, they came to the place where he was staying with the Witnesses and took him away. The killers took his body and put it in the river so that no one ever found it.

Another brother and sister were also killed. We heard rumors that they were dead, and then we never heard from them again.

Alfred Jallah, my father, was a chief in the town where we lived, with many wives and girlfriends: he had at least seventeen children, and maybe many more. In Africa, when a man is cheating on his wife, nobody gets so mad like they do in America. If the girlfriend comes around, we just accept her and the new children into the family.

My father was in so much danger that he was the first of our family to leave Liberia and get political asylum in the United States. He went to Boston from the Ivory Coast refugee encampment in Danané in 1994.

When the fighting started to come closer to where I lived in 1994, I sent my children to be with family members who lived in places not so dangerous. By then I had eight children, three boys and five girls. We could hear the soldiers coming, shooting everyone. Bam. Bam. Bam. People would be so frightened that everyone would run to jump in the river or hide in the swamp. One time, I was hiding behind a tree and the bullet went bam and then past my ear. I tried to make myself smaller behind the tree.

My aunt was in her house when the soldiers came and burned the house with her in it. When the soldiers left a place, everything would be gone. Houses. Food. Possessions. Children. No reason to come back. People would just start running from the soldiers and never return. The fear was so great that all anyone could think of was trying to stay alive.

Mothers would grab their children, but sometimes the children broke away and ran. Sometimes the mothers hid them someplace safe and kept running so the soldiers would follow them instead. Sometimes the children couldn't be found. Sometimes a woman would deliver a baby and then just get up and leave that child and run away. My grandmother was old and blind and couldn't run when the soldiers came. Everyone who was with her then left her when the soldiers were coming, and no one ever saw her again.

When you start running, maybe you have a little stuff, some food—two pieces of bread. No time to get anything—too hard to carry. If you see other people running, maybe you stay together, try to help each other. Every time we reached a good place in the bush, we would build a hut real fast. Rain would be coming down.

We would find branches of trees and cut sticks and put them in the ground. Then just put leaves up on the roof so it can't rain on you. After a day, you have to continue running. So you have to keep on, keep on, keep on. You don't know where you are going. Sometimes the soldiers see in the bush where you made a path and they follow to kill you. You are hiding, always hiding. You eat monkey fruit. You see something that looks like a fruit and see how it tastes. Then you eat it.

Maybe you trade what you found for another thing someone else has. Eat cassava root. One good thing is that God blessed Liberia with water. You drink from creeks, any kind of running water. It takes so long to walk. We are in this bush for so long, about a month. Finally we come to the Cavalla River, the border between Liberia and the Ivory Coast. With a little money I pay the boatman and he takes me over.

Eric and I came to Danané at different times. The Ivory Coast is a French-speaking country, but Gio, my family's tribal language is also spoken by many people. Eric and his family, who were from the Bassa tribe, came in 1991.

Eric went to a high school started by the Methodists. One of his relatives remembered that he was called the "tennis ball master" because he could make a tennis ball do anything he wanted, play it in any game. The boys were always wanting to play soccer, but they didn't have a soccer ball, just a tennis ball. Eric could hit the tennis ball with his head and body, kick it so well that it worked like a soccer ball. Nobody could play like he could.

He rode a motorcycle through the streets so fast that people would be afraid to ride with him. When Eric was in high school, he set up a phone booth so that people could call their relatives in the United States or Europe or other parts of Africa to ask for help. When some would come there without money in their pocket, he would say, "Go ahead and call, and when your money comes you can pay me."

Eric always helped people. If he was on his motorcycle and he saw someone who needed a ride, he gave them one. If someone needed money and he had some, he would give it to them. Everybody liked Eric. When he went down the street, people would be calling out his name, wanting him to stop.

When Eric was with people, he would notice how they were feeling. Maybe he would see from their face that they were unhappy. Then he would say, "What's wrong?" even if they hadn't said anything. He could just see their feeling.

Eric's family had been in Danané when it was a town with villages around it. By the time I arrived in 1994, many hundreds of thousands of Liberians were in the Ivory Coast.

Danané was a big city swallowing up all the little villages near it.

My aunt, who had a son in America, was living in Danané. This son sent her money so she was able to rent a house with four bedrooms where I could live with her. We used lanterns for light and we cooked outside on a wood fire. My aunt had a well that she dug. So we always had water. We were lucky to have such a big house.

Sometimes twenty-five people would be living in the house: refugees coming through, relatives, friends, and orphans. When people in my family saw people who had nothing, we would bring them home and make them comfortable until they could find their own homes. People used to laugh at me and say, "One day you are going to take a killer into your home."

I would say, "Well, that's how God made me."

At my aunt's house we would have people sleeping in the bedrooms, in the living rooms, in the hallways—everywhere. Then maybe some would leave and you would have a little privacy before new people came in.

To this day my aunt is still taking in orphans, calling me to say she needs money to help them. When I was in Danané, I helped take care of these children so much that my sister started calling me the children's slave.

When I got to Danané in 1994, I didn't know if my own children were dead or alive. Every day I would go out to buy phone cards. Nobody had phones in their houses. When we wanted to make calls, we would go to phone booths in the middle of town like the one Eric set up. But these booths didn't allow you to pay later. You had to buy phone cards that had maybe $5 of credit on them. Sometimes the operators would take so long that you would use up all your money before you talked to anyone.

Other times you would get a person to answer your call but it wouldn't be the one you wanted. So you would ask that person to tell your loved one to be back at the phone at a certain time, and you would call. Maybe you would be able to get through at that time, and maybe not. So I started calling everywhere I could think of to try to find my children.

Sometimes I would get someone in the town where my children had been living, and I would ask about my children, but all anyone could tell me was that they were gone. I kept calling whenever I had some money. Finally, one day when I called the town in Guinea where three of my daughters were, I got a man who said he knew my family. They were in the camp and he would tell them to call me. I waited by the phones all day the next day. No call. I waited the next day again, and then finally in the afternoon my daughters called. So that one day I wasn't worrying so much.

I also would ask everyone who came from Liberia if they had seen my children. One day I found a woman who was in Danané doing business; she went back and forth to Liberia. She had seen the rest of my children and told me that all of them were safe. In the next few months, my relatives arrived and five of my children were reunited with me. There was so much joy on that day. Only the three daughters in Guinea were still apart from me, and they were safe. I was very lucky.

I may have seen Eric before the day he called out to me on the road to the market. He lived not so far from my aunt's house. But I wasn't thinking about getting a boyfriend. So I didn't talk to him. I just kept walking like I didn't hear him. I was not thinking of having a man. I was always thinking of how to feed the five children I had with me. Every month we got food from the relief station, but it was so little.

Every day I would wake up before the sun came up, thinking in the dark, "Oh, God, how am I going to feed my children today?" Before it was even light I'd been thinking about how much food I had, where I might get more, and how long I should wait before cooking whatever I had.

My children might already be hungry when they woke up, but I could not feed them so early. I had to make the food last. If I cooked too early, they would be hungry and crying for food long before it was time for bed. So I would think every day about how long to wait and hope that they would keep sleeping. I always tried to wait until the morning was over and cook maybe in the afternoon so they wouldn't be so hungry before bedtime.

During the rainy season, making sure you had food was even harder. You would have to have your food inside the house before the rains started each day. Once they started, you couldn't go anywhere. The rain would be just flooding everything, and you would have to sit in your house and wait until it stopped. If you didn't have food, too bad. You just sat there, hungry, hoping the rain wouldn't last too long.

One day I was outside making a meal in the place where we cooked our food over wood fires. Maybe I was making potato leaf soup. I love potato leaf. Eric came over to me, talking and talking. He was wearing shades and nice clothes. He always talked about positive things.

"You look like such a nice woman. I wish you would talk with me," he said.

I told him that I did not need a man, but he wouldn't stop talking with me.

"I like you. I think I love you. Will you be my loved one?"

This talk did not surprise me. Some Liberians talk like that, lighthearted. They fall in love so quickly. And sometimes it lasts their whole lifetime.

My father fell in love with my mother just as fast. He worked on roads, telling the crews how to do the job. One day in one of the villages he was working in, he saw my mother. She had fallen in love with him, too. And so they married and were happy together. I heard all this from others. I barely remember my mother, who died when I was very young. I was raised by an aunt.

I was not too surprised to hear Eric say right away that he wanted me to be his loved one. I listened to him talk this sweet talk for a while.

Then I said, "Okay. I will talk with you."

I left the cooking to go over to talk with him under a flower tree. The next day, he came back and knocked on my door.

"Why don't you come outside and talk to me?" he said.

I was already liking him a little bit so I talked with him. He was a fine-looking man. He had hair then. This town of refugees was a place with lots of people who weren't happy, but Eric always was. He was joking and talking to me about happy things. Every day he came. I kept telling him that I didn't want a man.

He would say, "That's all right. I just like to talk with you."

I finally thought maybe I might fall in love with him.

When I was first with him, Eric was still being kind of a playboy. He said that life was so hard being a refugee in the

Ivory Coast that he had to keep enjoying his life. By enjoying his life, he sometimes meant enjoying other women. He would cheat on me. I would find out, and I would go to his parents' house, all mad. I would fuss at him and hit him on the head and the back and the shoulders.

He would just sit there with his head down and his hands on his lap. He wouldn't ever hit me back. He was always like that, not even raising his voice to me—always so respectful. After punishing him, I would leave for my own house. His mother would be saying, "Why are you hitting on my son?"

His sisters would say, "She is right to hit him. He's been cheating on her with other women."

He would sit there saying nothing even after I left. Another kind of man would be talking with his family about how bad I treated him. That kind of man would be lying maybe, making me look bad. Eric was always a gentle man. When people were all talking wild, Eric would be quiet. He would be waiting to make sure he didn't say any words that might be wrong.

After I left, he would wait a while, and then he would get up and start walking the way I had gone. His sisters would say to his mother, "Look. He's going back to his woman."

He would always be coming to my house at the end of the day. He would show up at the door, still looking so sad, and I'd let him in.

"I'm sorry," he would say, "but those girls are so tempting." I would be mad, but he was so sweet that I would forgive him. Nobody could stay mad at Eric.

Later he would say, "This shoulder of mine is hurting from where you hit me. You need to rub it." And I would.

Eric loved to come to my room. He was all the time just wanting to be with me alone. When we had food, we never ate with others. We went to my room so we could eat together. We would lie on the bed and talk and listen to music. All we liked was being together.

Eric was a quiet man but also brave. I learned this story while I was still in the Ivory Coast. When he and his family were running away from the soldiers in Liberia, escaping to the Ivory Coast, they walked many days through the bush just like I did. His mother had a little boy living with her, and that little boy went with them. In those days, the soldiers were kidnapping young boys. They were taking them into the armies and giving them guns and drugs, teaching them to do terrible things to people.

These boys were so young and so frightened that they would do anything for the people protecting them. Pretty soon these poor boys would not know what was right or wrong. Some of the terrible soldiers would even tell the boys that they were doing what God wanted them to do. God will judge them for that.

So when this boy that Eric's mother had with her went missing, everyone was afraid that he had been kidnapped and sold to the soldiers. People told Eric and his mother to forget about that boy. He wasn't even their relative. But Eric's mother could not stop crying for this boy. So Eric began to look for him. He searched for the boy for two years. It was dangerous even to ask about the lost boys, but Eric would not stop asking.

Eric loved his mother so much and never wanted her to get into trouble. He protected her. So Eric never told his mother he was searching for that child. He would go to the villages as if he were selling some things he'd brought. He would pull them out and show them to people, asking them to buy, but that was just his excuse to look around for the child. It was dangerous to ask directly.

He would stay and observe, going from house to house, going and looking and gathering information, but doing it in a very wise way. He would tell the story of the boy as though he were just talking. He would give the name of the boy and talk about the kind of boy he was, and when he had been last seen. But he would never say, "I am looking for that boy."

Finally, after two years of looking, he found the boy in a market. The boy had been found by another family that had taken him in and now considered him their son. So Eric went home and told his mother that he'd found the boy and that he was safe.

Eric's cheating was because of how much love he had. He loved me. He loved Karsiah. He loved his mother. He loved life. But a refugee's love can't root. It is always restless and can blow away. A refugee can have a house, but it cannot be his home. He is always hoping to go home or to immigrate somewhere else where there can be a future. A refugee is a man with no good job. He has no rights. Nobody respects him. Everything costs money. But a refugee has no way to make money. Somebody has to give him money. Maybe it's the United Nations or the Red Cross. Maybe it's his relatives in another country. He must always have his hand out.

When we were in Africa, cheating on me was Eric's only fault. I have to tell the truth about who he was. He was a player; otherwise, he was perfect. Sometimes men were fighting, but Eric never did. He gave me whatever money he had. Whenever anyone gave him anything, he would give it to me. I still woke up before it was light thinking about food, but now there was a warm man's body next to mine. I would put my face against Eric's back, both of us so skinny that it would be bone against bone with a little flesh between. He would turn over and put his arms around me. I would rest there in the only good moment of my day.

When I told Eric that I was pregnant with his child, he was so happy. He called my children his children from the beginning, but for us to have a child together was so wonderful to him. He talked all the time about how he would protect his son and what he would teach him.

I listened and continued to think about food. Where would I get it? How would I make it last?

Eric was always the cool guy. He never got into fusses; I was the one who did that. But what could I do when something was wrong? I had to say what I believed.

Here is one instance. When I was eight months pregnant, I was so tired that when the day came for us to get food, I couldn't walk to the distribution station. I gave my ticket to one of my daughters and told her to get the food for us. Every month the man at the distribution center got some oil, something like corn meal, some rice, and a few other things. If we didn't get this food, we would starve. When my daughter handed the ticket to the man who was giving out the food, he would not give her anything. He said that I would have to come myself. He took the ticket and sent her home.

I didn't have any choice. I had to get the food. So I came to the station with my big belly sticking out, so tired and now angry. I waited in the line for a long time with my feet hurting and that big baby pressing down. I was nervous about what would happen because I did not have the ticket now.

When I finally got to the front of the line, I told the man that I had come for the food he refused my daughter. He did not deny that my daughter had been there, but he wouldn't give me my food. He said that he had given the food to my brother.

I said, "My brother? What are you talking about? Show me which one you are calling my brother?" He said the man had gone.

"What is his name?" I said.

But the man had no name to give me. "He only told me that he was your brother, and you told him to get your food. Your food is gone," he said. "If you want it, go to your brother who has it."

This man was lying. I knew that he had given my food to someone who would sell it and then they would split the money. So I said very loudly, "Give me my food. You are keeping the food I need for my family."

But he wouldn't, and I didn't have our ticket. I was in a bad spot. All I could do was to keep calling for justice. So that's what I did. I kept telling him to give us our food. I would not move.

I just kept saying again and again, "Give me my food." He could not make me stop asking.

He went through the tickets until he found the one he had taken from my daughter. "Here, look," he said. "Here is your ticket. That shows that someone has taken your food. Go away."

But I would not, so he called a policeman.

"This woman is causing trouble and you must remove her," he said.

The policeman knew what that man was doing. Maybe he even had some share in it. Maybe he was going to get some money.

"You must leave this place," the policeman said. He did not care that my children would starve. "You are creating a disturbance. Other people are waiting to get their food."

He had a long stick he was beating through the air to threaten me. I could hear the swishing sound the stick made. My big belly was sticking out, and he was moving the stick closer to it, swinging it through the air, trying to make me afraid. But I would not move. I knew about this policeman; he was not a good man. People were watching and listening.

"I know about you," I said. "You hit a pregnant woman with that stick and she died."

No one had punished him for that. But I knew he did it. "Now you want to hit me with that stick and kill my baby. Get away from me with that stick. You need to hit that man who stole my food."

I said everything loudly so that other people would hear me and see if he hit me with the stick. He saw that people were watching, so he didn't dare to hit me.

But it was no use. I knew that the man who gave out the food would never admit that he sold my food. The policeman would not give me justice. What could I do? Refugees have no rights, but I was desperate. So I went to the office of the head of the refugee service, and I would not leave until he saw me.

I told him about how tired I was and about my daughter and how she was too afraid to ask for the ticket. He came back to the food station with me. He looked through the tickets. He found the one the man had taken from my daughter.

He said, "Give this woman the food for this ticket."

A few days later, I saw the man who had given my food away. I said to him, "God knows what you did. God will punish you for what you did, stealing my family's food."

Later I saw that man sitting with some other people. He said to them, "Don't mess with that woman. She cursed me before God. She is a dangerous woman."

After that I never had any trouble getting food.

The food that the refugee relief agency gave us at the first of every month was not enough. It lasted four, maybe five days. Sometimes we had no food at all, not even some greens to stir into water.

The month I was going to have Eric's baby, the food ran out, and I was without anything to eat for four days—no food at all. I was getting ready to have my baby and the midwife said, "You don't have the strength to have this baby. I have to get you some food."

So she went to some other people and asked them to give her food. They had just some greens. She stirred them in water and gave me the soup. I had my baby in the afternoon. I named him Eric Karsiah Duncan. Karsiah had been my grandfather's name and that is what I would call our son. My grandfather had died before I was born, but in the week before my son came into the world, I had a dream. In it an old man came walking into my house. He had a cane and white hair. He told me that my son was going to be a great man, very successful, a good man that many people loved.

I didn't recognize the old man, but when I told my aunt about the dream, she said that was my grandfather. We both knew what the dream meant. This son would be the rebirth of my grandfather.

I know that many people in America don't believe in dreams, but Africans do. We believe that dreams tell us what is going on in other worlds or sometimes in this world. We pay attention to the messages in dreams because they give us wisdom. I named Eric's son Karsiah to honor what the dream showed me, and Karsiah is turning out to be all that the dream said he would be. In the trouble that would come into our lives as Karsiah was turning nineteen, this boy would show judgment and wisdom. He would be the one who would lead me on a righteous path.

Eric and a friend had gone to another village on the day I had his son, but they came the next day, and he was so happy. He was so proud and talking so much and celebrating so much, walking about that room holding his son, that I finally had to say, "You need to stay out of the room because this baby needs to rest."

# CHAPTER THREE

## *Farewell, Liberia*

When I told Eric that I planned to cross the border back to Liberia, he begged me not to; but I was so scared of war. I said, "I'm not going to stay in this place that isn't even my home. If war is starting again, I'd rather go back to Liberia and die there."

The Ivory Coast was less dangerous than Liberia, but it was not completely free of violence. Soldiers came through recruiting men to go back to Liberia to fight. And when soldiers are around with different politics, there can be fights. But that wasn't all of it. So many Liberians were coming into the Ivory Coast that there were bad feelings with the Ivorians. They didn't want the Liberians taking jobs. If water or food was scarce, having the Liberians there made it worse.

When the Liberians would go into the bars to have a beer, fights would break out. Mostly it was just rudeness, but sometimes riots would start and were not easy to stop. People would get killed who had nothing to do with whatever the rioters were mad about. New things were always happening to provoke people. One big riot between the Liberians and Ivorians kept getting bigger and bigger. So I didn't want to be anywhere around. People were going so crazy and hating each other just like they had during the war.

I would do anything to get away from fighting. Eric could not protect me. "I just had a baby and if there is a riot, I can't run with my baby," I told him. "Your ways of thinking are not mine."

A few weeks after I had Karsiah, Eric and I parted. If he hadn't loved his son and me so much, that might have been the end of our story. But Eric always loved us and wanted us to be together. When we were apart, his love didn't get to be less.

I gathered all my children and went away with my sister. We paid a man with a boat to take us across the Cavalla River, back to Liberia. At first we lived in a mud hut in a village. I was used to living in a house made of concrete or brick, not mud. I slept with a flashlight and kept Karsiah next to me in the bed on one side, and the next-youngest child, Nopie, on the other. One night I thought I saw something crawling across the ceiling. It looked big enough to be a snake, but when I turned on the flashlight, I saw that it was a huge caterpillar.

If this caterpillar got on your face, people said it could get up in your nose and kill you. So I started screaming for my older son to come kill it. The next day I started putting rocks against the house where there were holes the insects could get through. I went around dabbing the walls where there were cracks. All day I was trying to keep the dangerous animals out, but at night I still couldn't sleep. The wilderness was right outside, with all sorts of dangers. I was afraid something would get in and kill my little children.

When my sister heard that I was sleeping in the day and keeping watch every night, she arranged for me to move to

a bigger house with better walls. In this new place, my children and I had a big room to ourselves, but we were alone,
which meant that animals could get into the other rooms.
No matter how hard I tried I couldn't get rid of all of them.
Right away I saw a scorpion. That night there was an insect
we call a "thousand legs." If it walks on you, every leg will
sting your flesh and leave a mark. So I was just as scared in
that house as I'd been in the mud hut.

"I don't know what I'm going to do with you," my sister
said.

"I don't know what I'm going to do with myself," I said. It
was clear that I liked a city better than the wilderness.

After a month, my sister went back to Danané to get
some soap and other things we needed for subsistence. Eric
saw her and gave her $40 to help us.

"Your sister has taken my baby away so that I can't see
him. I am sad all the time without them. I want them to
come back," he said.

But my sister spent the money on things we needed. I
can't say that I was spending all my time missing Eric. I was
too busy making sure the bugs didn't kill my children. But
hearing that he wanted me back did get my attention. When
a woman has a man who likes to run with other women, she
might need persuading.

Then my sister went to Danané again. Again she saw
Eric, again he said that he missed us. Again he gave her
$40. This time, he said, "Tell your sister to use this money
so that she can get across the river."

The riots had stopped and the dangerous insects were
still scaring me. Eric was offering a way. So I went back. Eric
was as handsome as a prince and all the girls ran after him.
But he wanted to be with me.

When I came back, he said, "We must get a place to live together."

But I said, "No. I don't want to live with you. My brother has a big house with four bedrooms. If I move out with you and you get tired of me, I'll have to leave and when I come back, my room will be gone."

So he would come to the house that my aunt's son paid for, where all my family lived. He would always bring gifts for the children and me. But when he brought something like a huge box of soap for us, kids would scatter it all over the house. People would use it so that there wouldn't be any for us. Again he said, "I want a place where you and our baby can live with me."

But I still said no; I liked things the way they were. "You have some of your clothes hanging where I live," I said. "You spend many of your days here. It's fine."

He said, "Okay, we will live how you say. When we get tired of living in your house, we'll go to mine."

And I said, "That's okay. That's very romantic."

On our baby's first birthday, we had a big cookout. All our relatives contributed food. We cooked yams and catfish. Eric loved catfish. My sister and I were in the yard dishing out food. There was music and lots of dancing. Eric brought his friends and carried his son around everywhere, showing him off. Even the Ivorians who lived next door came to the party.

When Karsiah was born, the Ivorians had come to dance outside our house. They said, "Oh, you have given us a new Ivorian man." From the very day he was born, people seemed to love Karsiah.

Eric and I might have gone on like that for many years. But my father was in Boston working all the time to get political asylum for his children. I was almost five years in the Ivory Coast when my visa to go to America came through. Everyone applied for an American visa as soon as they could, but it took a long time to get one and some people never did.

Eric and I sometimes talked of the life we would have together someday when we were both in another land, no longer exiles and refugees, but immigrants who could make homes they would be able to keep. America was the big dream. American movies. American music. American television. We loved kung fu stories with Chuck Norris, Jackie Chan, and especially, Bruce Lee.

Everyone knew about America. Lots of people had relatives there. These relatives had so much money that they could live in America and still send their African loved ones enough to live on. They had jobs that paid more money than we could possibly make. Americans were not hungry. They were not hopeless. We yearned to be in America. Whenever people got to go to America, they had a great opportunity. Those who stayed behind were sad to be left, but knowing someone in America was the next best thing to going there. If you knew someone, that person could send you money. That person could help you get to America.

In 1998, the US Refugee Admissions Program accepted me and sixteen of my brothers and sisters for political asylum. The word came that the US government would pay for our tickets to Boston, and that we needed to come to the offices to fill out papers. Eric was also trying to get political asylum, but he came from a different part of Liberia. The war had come there like it had come everywhere, but refugee status is difficult to establish. People would go to the UN offices again and again to try to get political asylum.

We would hear rumors and spend days and days at the United Nations trying to register. But you could spend the whole day there with nothing happening. Maybe the northern region where I came from was more recognized by the outside world as a place where killings were political.

Eric was happy for me, but we were also sad. The plan for everyone was to go whenever they could and bring their loved ones as soon as they could; this was in our minds. My going to America meant that we both had a chance. But we knew, as everyone did, that for those left behind, getting to America could take years—and that it might never happen.

I was thinking about Eric, but just as when I left the Ivory Coast to go back to Liberia, I was thinking more about my children than my man. I now had six children in the Ivory Coast and three in Guinea. Everyone knew that I could not take these children with me. People who admitted having children when they filled out the paperwork were denied a chance to immigrate. This was not a program for whole families.

My father had to go to America alone and now he was sending for his children. That was how it had to be done. Every day someone else would remind me that I must say I had no children. I would listen and say nothing. Their words made me too miserable to speak. Just about all the money we had to survive on came from Liberian family members who had jobs in America and sent us money. The only way for a refugee family to survive was to have family members in America. So even if you didn't want to leave your children, you had to. If you stayed with them, you would just watch them go hungry day after day and maybe die, with no doctors to help.

When I went to fill out the papers, I saw that a question asked if I had a husband. Eric was my husband. We hadn't gone to the church to be married, but everyone knew we were husband and wife.

This American program was not for husbands. If I said I wanted to bring a husband, I would not be going. I wrote, "None."

Then came the question "How many children?" I held my pen over that question for a long time. No official ever said, "You can't take your children." But everyone in Danané knew stories of parents who said they wanted to bring children when they filled out the papers: their papers were never approved. No one ever said what happened. The trip just didn't get made—no explanations. I knew that the right answer was zero children.

I sat a long time wondering if I could take at least the two youngest of my children. I had my first child before I graduated from high school. Almost all my life I'd had children snuggling against me at night, my own, my sisters', and my brothers'. My children were all I had. Karsiah was only two. He wouldn't remember me if I left now. I wouldn't be able to protect my children. I wouldn't see them grow up. I would be in America eating American food, not even knowing if my children were hungry. My heart pounded so hard that I could hear the blood in my ears. My body felt cold and so alone. A sadness fell over me that I would carry for the rest of my life.

Next to the line that said, "How many children will you bring?" I wrote, "None." Only a really terrible mother would stay in Danané because she was unwilling to make the sacrifice of leaving her children. I can never forgive myself for leaving my children. But to stay in the Ivory Coast would have been even more unforgivable.

In the weeks while I waited for my papers to be approved, Eric and I would sit every night on a long bench on the porch of his house. Karsiah and my little daughter Nopie would be with us, playing. Sometimes other people from our family would come to sit on the two steps that led up to the porch. One day my sister took a picture of Eric and the children with me on that bench. I have the picture but I never show it to anyone. It is an ugly refugee picture. I am so skinny and ragged and sad.

Eric was renting an apartment in a big house in Danané owned by a Frenchman. French people were not so nice to Liberians most of the time, but this one was okay. He let Eric rent from him. Unlike the house I lived in, this one had electric lights, but when we talked late into the night on the porch, we would keep the lights off so the big moths and beetles wouldn't come buzzing. Mosquitoes would be landing on our arms and faces, but we wouldn't want to go inside.

We wanted those last nights to last as long as they could. The air smelled of wood smoke from the cooking fires. The children would fall asleep, their heavy heads on our laps. We would talk into the night about how hard our lives were as refugees, and how much we wanted to go home. But going home was impossible. Refugees were still crossing the river with terrible stories. All that waited for us in Liberia was death. America was our only hope.

"If you send for me when you get to America, I will come and we will live together for the rest of our lives," Eric said.

I would laugh and say, "You will get to America and then abandon me for some other girl."

"I have lots of years," he told me. "Someday you will believe that you are the one true love of my life."

We both knew that I would be working every day to bring my children to America. As much as I loved Eric, he would be last on the list. But to say that would have been too mean. We would have been facing no hope. We always said that we were only parting for a little time. He would keep trying to get a visa. Maybe some of his relatives would get to America and send him a ticket to come. It happened all the time.

Before I left Africa, I had to think about where each of my children would go to live. Luckily, Africans have big families and many of my family were in Danané. My older children were able to find places to live with their friends or cousins. They were either ready to start their lives as adults or already had. The middle ones could stay with my aunt in the house her son paid for. Karsiah would live with my sister, and Eric's mother loved him so much that she would also care for him.

Karsiah's third birthday would be in September. My plane left in August. I wondered if there would be a big birthday party for Karsiah this year. Would Eric come with his friends and dance about the yard with his son in his arms? Would the Ivorians come again? I couldn't bear to think that he would have no party, and I couldn't bear to think that he would have one, and I wouldn't be there.

The day that the bus was to leave to take us to the Abidjan airport, we were very busy, getting transportation for me and my sixteen brothers and sisters, packing all the bags and making sure that we got to the bus. We were all getting something we'd dreamed about for years. All the other Liberians envied us. But no one was celebrating. Everyone was sad and crying.

I held each of my children for a long, quiet time so that I could remember how their bodies felt next to mine. My daughter Kebeh had tears running down her face. I kept wiping them away. Karsiah was too young to know what was happening, but the sadness was so great that he started to cry, too. Eric was with us. After a while, we just stood together without talking. There was no more to say. I waited until the last minute to get on the bus.

"You are going to have a wonderful life," he said. "We will be together."

I was crying, but he smiled at me. As I held him close one last time, I felt the new fullness of my breasts pushing against his chest. He hadn't noticed that my stomach, usually so lean, was just a little bit full. I walked through the gate, lonely but not really alone. I was carrying Eric's baby to America.

I had never been on a plane before. All of us were frightened. The plane was bouncing around, making terrible, clackety noises. We said, "Oh God, we're going to die." When the noises stopped, we were happy to be going to America but still so sad to be leaving loved ones. For many hours from light to dark and light again, we rode in the plane filled with air that was heavy and smelling like fuel, in clouds, over the water, going so far away, hoping never to return until we were rich enough to build a house where all our loved ones could live. We were the lucky ones. Sometimes being so lucky can feel good and terrible at the same time.

When we landed at JFK Airport in New York, we had to get on an escalator. We had never seen one. Everyone was pushing and stepping around each other, all in such a hurry and never looking at other people. An elderly woman who was with us was so scared when she looked down that long tunnel with sharp metal steps. She just froze up.

A man dodged around her and stood in front of her as others got on. She tapped him on the shoulder and said, "White man, please help me." He jumped like she'd pinched him.

Then he looked at her over his shoulder and said, "Get away from me."

Maybe this man didn't even know what she was saying. Everyone in Liberia speaks English, but it is British English, not American, and we speak it with our own accents. Adjusting to America is easier for us than many immigrants because we can read English better, but sometimes we can't understand American English, and often Americans can't understand us. So it isn't as easy as it seems. Americans can be irritated when they don't know what we're saying. Maybe this man was that way.

Laughing, we told the elderly woman, "We will help you. Just step on it." But she wouldn't. She was afraid.

So we all chanted, "Just jump. Jump." Finally she did. Holding onto the rubber railing she made it to the bottom.

The first meal I ever had in America was in the hotel restaurant, and it was so bad. My sixteen brothers and sisters and I all went together in our bright African clothes, with the women wearing African head ties knotted into headdresses. We stood tall and stayed close to one another. Many of the waiters looked alarmed at the sight of so many of us. They ran around looking for tables.

When we spoke to them, sometimes they didn't understand. So we learned to talk slowly, saying each word so that it was alone and clear. This was something we would be doing for a long time. Sometimes people would be angry that they couldn't understand us. They would yell, louder and louder. Maybe they thought that if they talked loud, they would be able to hear us better.

At our places on each table, we found cloth napkins with heavy knives and forks. It all seemed so fine. I ordered chicken. Liberians love chicken. When this chicken came it was so huge, bigger than any chicken I'd ever seen—and it wasn't even the whole chicken. I tasted the meat. It was soft—awful. I was hungry, but I couldn't eat this soft chicken that didn't seem like chicken at all. Liberian chickens are country chickens. They run in yards. They are skinny like the Liberians who eat them. They have meat that tastes like meat. It can be gnawed off the bone. This American soft chicken didn't have a bone. None of the Liberians could eat it, except one of my brothers.

"Give me your chicken," he said. "I am going to eat it all until I am very full. When you come to live in another place, you have to be willing to change what you like."

New York City was so noisy with horns honking everywhere. So many people were on the streets and all moving so fast. Nobody was just walking, enjoying themselves, having a good time greeting their friends. They didn't look at each other, just walked like they were late all the time. And so many people—where did all of them live?

Africans like to say, "Good morning," and to greet each other. But here no one was saying good morning. And so many people were wearing black clothes. Not smiling and in black, they looked like people who were very depressed. Africans like to wear colorful clothes with many designs.

And in Africa the sun is always shining. In New York, the buildings were so high and so many that the sun couldn't even reach the streets. I was glad we didn't stay there.

The next day we almost missed our bus to the airport because we had no idea how to get out of the hotel. The refugee people just took us there and left us. They took us to our rooms, but we went up the elevator and through the halls, around corners, and then we were there at our rooms. How did we get there? No one could remember.

Nobody showed us where they wanted us to be. They said, "Meet us at the bus." But where was the bus? We knew the time, and even though Liberians don't think about time very much, we all wanted to catch our plane. So we were ready on time. But where to go? How to find the right door? We just sat in our rooms worrying. What else could we do? We saw that time ticking away, but we were lost.

Finally, the refugee people realized that we weren't going to arrive at the meeting place, and they came to get us. We all grabbed our bags and went running as fast as we could. When we got outside, the charter bus was there, and the driver came out yelling, "Where are the African people?"

All the time I was thinking about how I would tell Eric these stories, and he would laugh. I would remember it all, and before he came to be with me, I would tell him how it really was in America. I would tell him to bring some African food of his own and to stay away from American chicken. As long as I kept saving these stories, I didn't have to admit that my man was really gone.

# CHAPTER FOUR

# *Making a Life in America*

When we got to Boston, our father was at the airport waiting with some other African people to welcome us. At his house where we would all live, there was lots of African food. Everyone had a party. They kept coming for two weeks to welcome us. It was so much fun, and I tried to remember it all so I could tell Eric. Then that good time ended, and we had to learn how to live in the real America.

All the houses in Boston look the same: the same color, all closed up, so many of them. We were afraid to go out. After two weeks I told my sister, "We have to get out of here and find our way around." We went out and walked down the street. We turned one corner and another and then we were lost. We looked and looked for something familiar. But every block looked just like the other one.

We walked and walked, looking for where we lived. What were we going to do? In Africa, we could have stopped at any house and told the people there our father's name. Someone would have known him in that house or the next one. People would have been out on the streets, talking and getting to know each other. We could have asked for our father and just kept asking until someone knew him—but not in Boston. In Boston, nobody knew who their neighbors were. People on the streets were all going somewhere. They didn't stop and visit with each other. We could wander around forever and never find our father's house or anyone who knew him.

My sister said, "You are the cause. We were in the house and then we come out and get lost."

"We have to keep walking," I said. What else could I say? It was my fault and I didn't know how to fix it. But then a miracle happened. I looked and there was our house number. We were so grateful that we fell in the door laughing, and we both thought that we would not go out ever again.

Even though I was in America, I still had to go to a phone booth to make calls. It was as hard to get to Africa as it had been to call America. Sometimes I called two, three days before I could leave a message. I told my sister in Africa, "Can you tell Eric to call tomorrow so I can speak to him?"

I went to the telephone booth the next day and waited for the call. When I got him, finally, I didn't have any good stories to tell. He seemed so far away—in another world. In the Ivory Coast we had always been face to face, never just a voice.

"Everything is okay. I miss you," I said. "This is a different place. You can't go outside. It's so boring. We just watch TV."

"Do you miss us?" he asked.

"Yes, so much I miss my son. I go in the bathroom and cry. I miss you so much."

"I come to your house," he said. "I look around your room and I don't see you. I look at our son and miss you a lot."

These conversations didn't always make me feel better—maybe worse. I would be all excited to hear Eric's voice, and afterward I would want to cry again. I wanted him to come to me, but this life in America was so hard. Not hard like refugee life, but hard in different ways.

Before September ended, I thought I was going to freeze to death. It was so cold that I cried. All the people who had been in Boston for a while laughed and laughed. "This isn't even cold. Wait until winter comes," they said.

The Liberians who had been there for a long time laughed loudest. They said I must get tough.

I had never been in a place that wasn't hot. I'd heard about snow, but I had never seen it. And ice: how could we know about walking on ice? We had never seen such slippery ground. My brother slipped on the ice and broke his leg. I also fell and hurt my leg.

When we arrived, we didn't have coats. Our shoes were not boots. Lucky for us, the charities brought us many clothes: big heavy shoes and socks, sweaters that itched against your skin, and coats. I'd never seen such big coats. I wore dresses in Africa, but in Boston the wind comes up a dress until every part of you is shivering. I put on so many clothes that I could hardly move my arms.

I was aching for my children, my heart swollen with pain. I wished every night that I had Eric to hold me as I fell asleep, and to kiss me when I woke up. I remembered how happy he had been dancing with Karsiah on his first birthday. Having Eric's baby inside me gave me someone of my own. In Boston everything was dead and frozen. But inside me was something warm and alive. I didn't tell anyone about the baby.

I was so lonely and so cold. I told Eric, "If you come to America during the cold time, you don't feel like you're on earth. You don't feel like you're a human being."

He seemed so far away. I missed Africa so much: the hot sun; the laughter of neighbors coming through the windows from the yards next door. I wanted the earth beneath my feet, not concrete. I wanted to live on the ground, not in a big dirty building where people never see each other.

No one in America could find a quick way to get some food. If you wanted to stir some leaves in water for a soup, you had to find a place to buy even a handful of leaves. No one would ever think of knocking on their neighbor's door to ask if they have some food to share. People in Africa were poor, but on the beautiful beaches and in the rivers of Liberia, people could catch fish, and in the jungle anyone could hunt animals.

I remembered how my son would take his dog to the bush and hunt animals for our dinner. He had such a good dog that they always came home with something good. I missed the palm trees that gave us palm oil. I missed the green of the bush and the air that smelled fresh. And most of all I missed the freedom to saunter down the street, hearing some music from the radio and dancing because I wanted to. Africans don't think it's strange if someone wants to dance, but in Boston I never saw anyone dance.

I missed the soft sound of Africans speaking English. I missed being in a place where people came and went by their own time, not always looking at the clock. And maybe most of all I missed being able to sit outside without being afraid that someone was watching and would do something bad to you.

When I went outside I couldn't see the bodies of people at all. Their faces were covered and so were their hands. Everybody was moving so fast so that they wouldn't freeze. The first time my hands got so cold that my finger wouldn't work, I was terrified. When I tried to touch anything with those frozen hands, it hurt more. Inside the houses even, it was always cold. I wanted to pile blankets on myself and never leave the bed. But I could not do that. When my brothers and I moved into a place of our own, my brothers were so afraid that we couldn't pay our bills that they told me not to turn on the heat. So we lived in a place where everything was freezing, including the water. And the food didn't even need to be in the refrigerator. I was just dying from the cold outside and inside until my father came to see me. He told my brothers to stop letting it get so cold. We would just have to work harder so that we could pay our bills.

In America everything was work: work, work, work. Get up, shower, eat fast, go to work, come home, sleep, get up, shower, eat fast, and go back to work. No time for anything else. My father told me, "In America, you must work to survive."

In Liberia, I always had good men who worked to support me and my children. I didn't go to school enough to be capable of getting a job. I didn't really think about getting one. I lived on my men. In our culture, men take care of us. If a man wants you, he's got to take care of you.

In the Ivory Coast there was no work for Liberians, so no reason even to look for work. But in America everyone had to work.

The refugee people gave us classes on how to live in America. They told us about going to work and about being on time. One thing I learned about America is that time is so important. Everyone is looking at time, measuring time, saying "There is not enough time." Being on time was important in everything.

I'd been a little bit prepared for this by a dream I had before I left Africa. In this dream, my brother told me that in God's new order everyone would be on time. He said being on time would prepare me for it. Maybe this made America's attitude about time seem a little more reasonable for me.

I got a job at a hotel with a fast-food area. It was so busy. Manager calling you to clean the bathroom, take out the trash, paging you on the phone, "Come upstairs," as soon as you got there. "Come downstairs."

"I have to leave this job," I told the manager. "You need me everywhere at once. I can't do this. I have to leave." Six dollars an hour is maybe a good wage in Africa, but in America the bills are very high. There is plenty of food to eat and lots of places to live, but everything is expensive.

When I told the manager I was leaving, he didn't believe it. He said, "Can you stay until the end of the hour?"

I said, "That's too long for me."

When I got home, my daddy said, "How you going to pay your bills? You can't quit your job."

I started to cry: "Why did people lie to us about America? We thought it would be good, but this is so bad. All we do is work." I was thinking, *I can't make it. This is too much work. You are always watching the clock.*

My daddy said, "You have to get used to it."

The refugee people got my sister and me a job processing food for restaurants. Every morning we would get up while it was still dark. I was so afraid of not getting up on time that I could not sleep. I'd be all the time waking up to check the clock. Someone told me to use an alarm. That helped. We took three buses and three trains to work. Sometimes we would go to work and they would say, "Go away. There is no work today." So we would turn around and travel three hours to go home. No work, no money.

One time I had to speak: "Why you don't call us to tell us, 'You don't come in today'? It would it be better if you let us know."

The manager apologized and said they would. That made it better, but still this job didn't always have enough hours to make our trip worth it. The work was hard.

We were in a big warehouse with about a hundred people working in shifts. There was a kitchen area where people were frying and baking. To us, the only two Africans in the building, they gave the worst job, cutting onions. They would bring big sacks of onions, hundreds of pounds that we would have to peel and chop. Our tears would come running down our face. People passing by would make fun of us. They would go away laughing. Sometimes we would get lucky and be chopping carrots, bell peppers, tomatoes, lettuce. We didn't stop peeling and chopping for as long as we were there, but still we didn't make enough money to live.

I told my sister that we had to quit.

She said, "No. The refugee people got us that job. They will be mad at us."

The refugee adviser said, "That food manager loved you and likes how much you work."

I said, "I thank God for you. What you've done for us. But I have to look for my own job. I did not come to America to be loved. I came to make money to support my children. I can't put love in an envelope and send it to my kids. I have to have more money."

I came to America for a better life and I would work for that. But in America, I found a new kind of hard time. No children. No man to love me. And now I knew that I must lose the one happy thing in my life; I must abort my baby. America is too hard for a single woman with a baby.

A single woman with a baby can't work enough. Everybody in the family must work. No one can stay home to care for children. No neighbors can watch them while they play. This is a place where no one will even give you a ride. So who would watch a baby? Who would fix my food until I got back on my feet? Who was going to pay my bills?

I had nine children in Liberia. Always they were welcome and cared for. I never thought about having an abortion. My nine children lived through war and exile and hunger. They lived in Liberia with danger everywhere. They ran from war to refugee camps where everyone treated them badly. They lived in hard places. But we all survived.

I remember how happy Eric was when he knew I was going to have Karsiah. I remember the Ivorians coming to dance outside my house when they heard that Karsiah was born. I remember Eric dancing with our son when he was one year old. Now all my children were far away from me, and this baby could not be born.

I waited a month with that baby growing, knowing more and more what I had to do. Then I found the clinic where they gave abortions. I had to do it. If I didn't work, my Liberian children would never have good lives. They would be exiles always. I thought of the faces of each of my Liberian children when I lay deep in the blankets trying to stay warm at night. I had come to America for them.

I told my sister I was not feeling well: would she go with me to the clinic? She went with me and waited while I had the abortion. I didn't tell her what I'd done until we were going home. She said, "Why didn't you tell me?" There was no reason to tell her because no one could help. I was grateful she came with me; then we were both sad.

Afterward, I regretted it; I cried that I had done something like that. I wondered if I could have found some way to keep the baby. But I had to accept it. I was happy then that I had not told Eric about his baby.

When Eric called, his voice was so welcome. I was sad and tired, and he would always be cheerful. He'd say, "I love you, sweetheart. Don't forget about me. We will be together someday."

We lived in Dorchester where there was so much crime. I had two jobs, one in the day and one at night, a security job at a hospital. Once coming late, I saw a bus coming, the kind of little bus Mexican workers ride in, going real slow. Some cars came and it went faster. Then it came back, driving like it was hunting me. I prayed and prayed, "God help me. God help me."

We weren't supposed to go on other people's porches, but I got to a porch and lay down so the driver of the bus couldn't see me. Then I ran to the road in front of the cars and to my door, banging on it. My sister opened it and I fell into the room.

"Go look out the window," I said to her. "You will see the bus." So she did and there it was.

Another time I was going to work very early in the morning in the dark and a brown car stopped. A man in a mask got out of it and came toward me like he was going to grab me. But just then another man came walking fast up the street, and the man in the mask ran back to his car and drove away.

"Did you see that guy?" I asked the man who walked up.

"Yes. That's why I walked so fast," he said.

I thought, "I can't work like this. I can't go to work so early and so late. I'm not going to risk my life for a job."

I heard that a nursing home needed nurses' assistants. The Red Cross would pay to train them. I signed up. There were thirty in our class. Only twelve graduated and I was one of them. Work at the nursing home was hard, but it was more human. If you needed a break, you could take one to get a little water or a soda. People cared a little bit about how you felt. They wanted you to work but also to have a little break if you needed it.

The pay was so low that I still had to work two jobs. One day I had been working the night shift, and they asked me to work one extra hour. So I did. On the bus I was so tired that I fell asleep. I woke up when the bus stopped and the driver came back to see why I had not gotten off. We were at the end of the line far away from my house.

"What are you doing here?" the bus driver said.

"I missed my stop," I said, so tired still, and not even knowing where I was.

"Let me smell your mouth," he said. He thought I might be drunk. But when he could tell that I had no alcohol on my breath, he said, "I will take you home." So I was able to make it to my house.

I wanted Eric to be with me. I missed him every day. But Africa was far away, another continent. I knew we might never be together again. I had no extra money. I sent everything I could to feed my children. And so I went on with life, just working, too tired even to dream.

I first talked to Peterson Wayne when he called on the phone for my brother. I delivered the message. Then he called again for me to give another message to my brother. I gave him my brother's phone number and said not to call me again. But after a few days, he called again and I picked up the phone.

"Didn't I give you my brother's number?" I said.

"I just called to say hi," Peterson said. I could tell from his voice that this man was also from Africa.

When he called again, I thought, "I got a man over there in Africa. So I don't want to talk to this man." I changed my number.

Then after a year, Peterson called me again. I said, "Who gave my number to you again?" He called my father and my brothers until he got it. This guy had never met me. He said, "I just love your voice."

"I don't need a man," I told him. "I got somebody."

"Where?"

"In Africa," I said.

"Africa is a long way off," he said.

"But that's where I came from, and somebody there is waiting for me," I said.

I had been in America about a year. I was lonely, but Eric was my man. We still talked, and we still thought maybe he would come to America.

Then something happened that caused us to give up on each other. I asked Eric to help my brother's children go to the interview for immigration. He didn't do it, and they missed their appointment. This was so serious because they might not get another chance. My brother was so disappointed and afraid that his children would never be able to come now. I was so angry with Eric. I was remembering that he didn't always do right. He knew about visa interviews, but he made my brother's children miss their chance.

I called him and I said, "You didn't help me." He knew just what I meant. So he was all defensive.

"You don't pay my rent," he said.

"Oh, I see," I said. "You can't do me a favor? You don't care to help me?"

I was so pissed off, thinking he was worthless. I was thinking that he would for sure leave me for some other girl if he ever came to America. I was all mad and piling up everything bad about Eric in my mind. So the next time Peterson called, I did not talk about my man in Africa. I told Peterson that maybe we should meet. And so we got together. He was a working man, a security guard.

I didn't call Eric again. But lots of phone calls were going back and forth to Africa. It wasn't long before Eric heard that I had a boyfriend.

He said, "Why should I wait for someone who is not faithful to me?"

I heard that he was saying this, but I didn't care. It wasn't long before Eric got a girl and got married. They didn't stay together, but by the time they split, I was already leading my own life.

Peterson and I fell in love. He said he would take me to Dallas, Texas, a place much warmer. I was in love with this man, yes, but for sure I was also in love with not being so cold. When he left for Texas, I went with him.

In Dallas we found the Liberian community. Lots of Liberians were living in Vickery Meadow, a place with many blocks of apartments. No houses painted blue or pink like in Africa. Not many trees. We found an apartment there, and at least Dallas was not as cold as Boston. I liked that. But the city, I didn't like.

Everyone was living in buildings with only parking lots around them. Our apartment seemed big, with many rooms. But no people—just us. So lonely. Nobody was on the streets at all. Nobody walked anywhere. Just cars everywhere. People always in their cars going fast, worrying about time. Honking. Speeding.

I found work in a nursing home. The pay was so low that I couldn't believe it. This work was hard and dangerous and sometimes nasty. Emptying bed pans. Picking up big people, people bigger than me who are so heavy—and I carry them by myself. Some don't help at all and stay limp while I am struggling to keep them from falling. Some act so mean.

Most of the elderly are all right. Some are grateful, so sweet. Mostly the mean ones are children who don't take care of their own elderly. They don't keep them. So I take care of them. I understand. Maybe they can't take care of their own loved ones. But I am sometimes thinking that they could be nice to me, the one taking care of their elderly. That's not too much.

At first I won't do this work for so little money, $6 an hour. But no jobs pay more. So I take the job. Years go by and I am working, and then I get maybe a dollar more an hour and then a dollar more than that.

In 2001, I had my American son, Timothy, delivered at Texas Health Presbyterian Hospital Dallas, the closest one to our apartments. In the American way, I stayed home with him only a month and a half before I went back to work. In

2006, I got permission from the Immigration Department to bring Karsiah to live with me. He was ten, a skinny little boy who didn't remember me at all. He stayed with my sister all those years, going from refugee camp to refugee camp. The camp was far away from where the phone booths were located. So I had not even talked with Karsiah much during the seven years since I left.

When I knew he was coming to be with me, my sister brought him to the phone.

I told him, "I am your mother. I love you so much, and you are coming to be with me in America."

I was just a voice to him. He didn't know about America. When he came here, he was so confused. I was overjoyed to welcome him. The day he arrived with Nopie, Youngor, and Joejoe, Youngor's younger son, then about two, I stayed home from work to cook African food to greet them. Peterson Wayne picked them up at the airport. When I went out to the car, I embraced Karsiah and said, "I'm your mother."

Then I told the others, "Here is my little grandfather," because he is named for the grandfather who'd come to me in a dream.

To Karsiah, it didn't feel like a better life because he was used to other ways of living: no school, always outside playing with other children, and lots of people around all the time. I was a stranger to him in a strange place. But one thing Karsiah did love right away is that school is free. He did not go to school regularly in the refugee camps because school cost money, and there wasn't enough to pay for education.

In the Dallas public schools, they put him in fifth grade so that he would be with kids his age. He didn't know fifth-grade work. He couldn't read well, and he didn't know history or science. Americans had a hard time understanding his accent. But they put him in English as a Second Language classes. He had a hard time at first. What he says is that it wasn't so bad because other Liberian kids were trying to learn, too. Karsiah is a cheerful, optimistic person like Eric.

I don't remember it the same way. I remember kids throwing rocks at him and calling him a little African monkey. But he stood up to them. He'd fight them. Finally, they got tired of fighting with him and started making him a friend.

At first, Karsiah was unhappy with me. We didn't know each other. He said I was too hard on him. I made him study. I told him, "This is not refugee camp. This is America. You are not here to play around. You must study and learn." But he was always a well-trained boy, and he did what I told him. "When you go to school," I told him, "work hard and people will help you."

His teacher made him partners with a boy in a wheelchair. I was not so happy about this because I thought it would make Karsiah be apart from the other children. But Karsiah did not complain. He made friends with the boy in the wheelchair, and he made sure everything was going well for his new friend.

Karsiah was just like Eric, always smiling. People at the school said, "That boy smiles so much; he probably smiles even in his sleep." Everybody loved him. They still talk about him at his schools. He was so smart and so happy to get the chance to learn. So soon he caught up with the other students.

All that playing in the refugee camps must have some value because anytime they give Karsiah a ball, he can play with it. If they give him a soccer ball, he can be on the soccer team. If they give him a baseball, he can throw it.

Eric and I talked some before Karsiah came to Dallas, but once he came to live with me, we had more reason to talk. People were starting to get cell phones and calls weren't so expensive. Eric would call more and more, and we would talk about our son. Karsiah hadn't grown up with Eric. His only memory was of one day when he was at his grandmother's house in Danané and Eric came by riding a motorcycle. Maybe Eric had been there many other times, but it was his father on a motorcycle that the little boy remembered.

Their conversations were not easy. Karsiah could not understand Eric's accent. And Eric could not understand Karsiah much better. Even though Karsiah had been in Africa until he was ten, our son had learned to talk more like an American. Sometimes Karsiah would say, "You have to talk with my daddy and tell me what he has to say." Eric would say that every time he talked to Karsiah, his son would be quiet: "All I hear is 'uh-huh.'"

Karsiah explained to me, "I say 'uh-huh' because I cannot understand the man."

So I told Eric, "Your son says it's hard to understand you. You need to go slow in talking to him. And speak louder."

Whenever he spoke to Karsiah, Eric would always say the same things. Study hard. Do right. Obey your mother. You are lucky to be in America. Karsiah didn't say much back, but he understood those messages.

Karsiah studied hard and he grew big. Peterson Wayne, his stepfather, liked watching basketball and Karsiah watched with him. He started to think that he could play the game. In middle school, he got on the basketball team. Karsiah was good at basketball and good at making friends.

His studies were going well by then, too. And Karsiah was so popular. Kids texted him all the time. His basketball coach at Conrad High School said he fit in like every other kid but was calmer and more polite with adults. Always sweet, just like Eric. He was co-captain of the basketball team. He ran track. When Karsiah was in the eleventh grade, a coach asked him to try playing football. Karsiah was six foot three and 190 pounds. The coach didn't plan to give Karsiah such a big role. He hadn't played football before.

But one day the coach saw him throwing a football with his teammates. Karsiah can throw a football hard and fast. He can make it go wherever he wants. The coach made him a quarterback. College scouts started watching him.

In one game, Karsiah's team was losing 18–7. Karsiah said, "Coach, put the team on my back, I got this." He made five touchdowns. His team won 42–32, and Karsiah was a hero of the school. Our son had lots of trophies, and his closet was full of athletic shoes. His coaches say he is a tremendous all-round athlete and leader. In spring of his senior year at the Texas Christian Athletes of the Year banquet, Karsiah won the courage award. This award was for the whole state.

Eric called often in those years and always he would say, "Let me speak to my son." Most of the time Karsiah would be practicing or playing a game or studying. I'd say, "Your son is a busy boy. He doesn't have time to talk with you." But sometimes they would talk.

Once, after Karsiah had graduated from high school, he had a summer job working in a warehouse to make money for a car. Ebola was starting to break out in Liberia and people were protecting themselves by buying bottled water. Eric needed money for the water. So he asked Karsiah to send him $50. But I needed Karsiah's money for the light bill.

"I must have that money or they will turn off the lights," I told Eric. And so Karsiah gave the money to me. But the next week when he was paid, Karsiah took $50 and sent it to Eric. Karsiah knows about the poverty of living in Africa. He was happy to help his father.

"I am so impressed with this son of mine," Eric said.

Karsiah is good in every way. When he was in high school, he had no girlfriends that he introduced to me because he had to finish his studies and make money before he could have a girlfriend. He thought all the time about doing well in school. When Eric would call, sometimes every day, to talk to his son, he would often talk to me. During our years apart, Eric had other women in his life, of course. He had three other children by then. But he never stopped telling me I was the love of his life. "You are the mother of my son," he would say. "You are my wife."

He did not care that I was married to another man and also had a son with that man. He and I were married, Eric said, and we always would be. I did not encourage this talk, but I understood it. In Africa, when a woman and a man have a child together, they are more than husband and wife. Sharing a child makes them always joined.

At the time Karsiah was ready to graduate from high school, Eric had been in Liberia for some years. The neighborhood in Monrovia where he lived some as a boy had been bombed. Now it was poor. Eric had also lived at

missions when he was a boy. I had been living at missions
some, too, when I was a child. Many were gone now. Liberia
was a lovely little country before the war. Now so much is
ugly.

Eric gave up on getting an American visa in the Ivory
Coast, and he was tired of so many French people being so
mean. He'd moved to Ghana, where he thought it might
be easier to get a visa. It wasn't Liberia, but people spoke
English. Things had gone a little better in Ghana. He went
to school and learned to be a mechanic. He studied computers and opened a little store that sold groceries. Oliver
Smallwood, one of his nephews, came to live with him and
helped him with the store. Even as a young boy, Eric had
been industrious. At age eleven in Liberia, he was harvest-
ing palm oil from trees and going to Ghana with family
members to sell it.

But Eric didn't get an American visa in Ghana, either.
When the war was over in Liberia, I told Eric, "You might as
well go home. It might not be better. Maybe you won't get a
visa there, either, but at least you will be home." And so he
went back to Liberia in 2012.

He still wanted to come to America, but he had no luck.
In Liberia, the American Embassy is like a hill, one many
people wish to climb. But to get a visa, someone in America
has to sponsor them.

"I want you to help me. I am desperate to come that
way," Eric told me. But I had no legal relationship with Eric
that would help.

"There is nothing I can do," I said. "The only way for
you to get to America is through your son." A relative has
to bring someone to the United States, and Eric and I were
not formally married. Karsiah was the link.

# CHAPTER FIVE

# *The Day He Didn't Call*

In the two weeks before he left Monrovia, Eric called me every single day—except one. I don't remember which day it was, although I often wondered about it later. Was that the day that Eric heard cries of "Help me, help me," coming from his landlord's house?

Late hours could not be the reason he failed to call that day. Sometimes Eric called so late at night that he woke me up. I need to sleep so I can go to my work as a certified nurse assistant at a senior living center. I told him I was going to turn off my phone if he didn't stop calling at night.

He said, "Oh, please don't turn off your phone. When I want to talk with you, I have to call. Please just wake up and talk to me."

It was so important to him that he talk to me that he would call no matter the hour. But he said nothing of the day that changed our lives forever. Why? Maybe it is because he was so eager to leave the life of his past; we did not talk of Africa. For us, even the present was not of consequence. The future we would make together was everything; it had been so long delayed. We talked every night about how our life would be when he came to Dallas. We had many plans.

He would get a job driving a big truck, an eighteen-wheeler, something he had done before in Africa.

"When I get there, I will work hard. Together we will work and have enough money," he said. We would save our money. And when there was enough, we would send it to Liberia for a house to be built. When that house was built in maybe two years, we would go back to Liberia and maybe we would live there, he said. I hadn't thought I would ever return to Africa. All my money goes for rent and bills and food and back to Africa for my loved ones. But Eric loved to work. In America, such a man can do well.

These plans didn't seem real to me at first. But Eric kept talking.

"You will see your three sons and their wives and children. They all love you so much," he told me on the phone.

I listened, and these ideas started growing in me. In Liberia we would start our own business, Eric said. We would buy some cars and hire some drivers. We would be able to build a good life. Always he was positive.

If I would tell him of my troubles, he would always say, "When I get there it will be better."

In the weeks before he came, when a whole day and night went by and he did not call, I was surprised. I was suspicious. Maybe he had another woman and had spent the day comforting her because he was going to leave. When he called the next day, I accused him of this.

He said, "No, sweetheart. You must stop having these bad thoughts and be positive. I am not that kind of man anymore. I have no other woman. You are my only love."

Now that our life together has ended, I wonder if the day Eric did not call me was September 15, four days before his plane left Liberia. I found out what happened that day from newspapers, from my son who investigated it, and from a relative of the people it happened to.

On September 15, Eric was coming home from work to the small room he rented in Paynesville, a town east of Monrovia. In his neighborhood, the little houses are painted green, blue, and pink. The earth around them is sandy. In Africa people are outside their houses a lot, so everyone knows what's happening in the neighborhood. To go to the house where he rented the room, Eric had to pass his landlord's house. He heard his landlord, Emmanuel Williams, calling, "Help me, help me!"

Eric went inside the house. Most people's doors are open in Liberia, so he didn't have to knock. Marthalene, the landlord's daughter, was nineteen and seven months pregnant and very sick. This was a girl who was always moving around, very restless. Everybody knew that she couldn't stay still.

But now this girl was not moving around at all. She was so weak she could hardly even raise her head. Her father said something was wrong with the pregnancy. He had called an ambulance, but Liberia had a lot of Ebola. Thousands of people had died already and many more were in hospitals. So maybe all the ambulances were busy.

When no ambulance came, the landlord called a taxi. He asked Eric to help get the girl into the taxi and to help them get to a doctor. Sonny Boy Williams, Marthalene's brother, who was two years older, helped, and so did Eric.

Eric sat in the front seat of the taxi. The other two held the girl in the backseat. Many people give different accounts of what happened next. It seems that they went to the Blessing

Home Clinic and two hospitals looking for help. Some people say the girl was vomiting. Some people say she vomited
on Eric. Some say she was bleeding from the mouth. But
these stories came from people who weren't there.

Afterward, everyone was so scared that they had all sorts
of stories. Here is one thing that seems clear: when they got
home, nobody in the car said anything that made anybody
think Marthalene had Ebola. At the Blessing Home Clinic,
they said she had malaria. Nurses put her on an intrave-
nous drip. But she kept getting worse and started having
convulsions. She needed a hospital. When they took her
to the John F. Kennedy Hospital hoping to get into the
pregnancy ward, she was turned away. Some reports say she
was also turned away at some hospital Ebola wards because
there were no beds.

People in Liberia get sent to the Ebola ward even when
they don't have Ebola. People won't go to hospitals at all because even when they have some not-serious illness, doctors
will put them in the Ebola ward. Even if they didn't have Ebola when they went in, they will get it while they are there.
So nobody knows how many people who don't have Ebola
would not get it if they stayed away from the Ebola wards.

What I do know and what everybody says is that in Eric's
neighborhood there were no cases of Ebola at that time.
Later, neighbors said the Williams family hid the girl's true
condition. Some said the family told everyone that their
daughter had malaria, that they even bought malaria pills
from a local nurse. Others said the family claimed she had
low blood pressure and died from pregnancy complication.
Other neighbors even said the family told people Marthalene had been in a car accident.

No one knows what the men said in the taxi that day. They drove all around Monrovia and waited for hours to be helped. Then they gave up. That evening when Martha-lene was brought home, she could not walk. Sonny Boy supported her torso, her father held her arms, and Eric held her legs so they could carry her across the sandy yard into the family's house.

Some people say she died in the taxi with the baby coming out of her. Other people say they placed her on the floor of the living room, and she died the next morning with all her family around her crying. They straightened her body, curled up from all the pain. Then they made her ready to bury. When a woman dies in childbirth, Liberians bury her that day. It will bring bad luck if they don't. People who loved her washed her and covered her. The landlord asked neighbors to help lift the body into her casket. Some people were afraid, maybe, but they couldn't refuse the father.

When someone in Liberia dies with Ebola, the body is burned. This girl was buried, so no one suspected that she had Ebola. About a hundred people came to honor her.

I don't know if Eric went to the funeral; that was the week for him to be packing for his trip to the United States. I told him not to bring many clothes because we could get clothes, and he could wear some of his son's extra clothes. But Eric was a churchgoing man, and he wanted to make sure he had good clothes for Sunday services. He filled a black rolling suitcase with brightly colored shirts, some with African patterns on them, khaki pants, jeans, underwear, and the nice gowns that African men like to wear. We call them gowns; Americans say they are caftans.

In a satchel he would carry onto the plane, he put his passport, his visa, and his United Air plane ticket. I read that he told one neighbor that he was going to America and would return in two years to build his own house. Another story said he told a friend that he was going to marry a girl in Dallas. Another man remembered him talking about a son who played baseball. At 11:00 a.m. on Friday, he left for the airport.

At Monrovia Airport Eric's temperature was taken as he entered the parking lot. It was taken again before he was allowed into the airport. It was taken again at the gate. Each time it measured 97.5. He was also asked whether he had been in contact with anyone who had Ebola or if he had touched the body of anyone who had died of Ebola. He said no.

When he was asked to fill out a form that asked the same questions, he wrote down "no." He was allowed to board the plane. His flight would stop in Brussels. He would change planes, go to Washington, DC, change planes again, and finally arrive at Dallas–Fort Worth International Airport the next day.

Eric was gone from Liberia before anyone in his neighborhood died of Ebola. But at about the same time Eric began to get ill in Dallas, Marthalene's brother Sonny Boy, who had been in the backseat of the car with his sister, also became ill. He died on the Wednesday before Eric went to the hospital emergency room. The neighborhood in Paynesville soon filled with ambulances, body collectors taking away the dead, and health officials looking for people with symptoms. Sarah Smith lived in the pink house next door to the Williams house. She died. Marie Wread had taken care of Sarah Smith when she was sick. She went to the hospital in an ambulance, looking very ill. Neighbors were so scared that they put her little daughter, Mercy, who was not sick, in the ambulance with her.

Marthalene's parents, Emmanuel and Amie, were admitted to the Ebola ward. Amie died. Emmanuel is still living. I heard that nine people died in all: ten in the end. Maybe Eric did not tell me of helping this girl because she died in childbirth. Maybe he did not want to remind me of my own daughter who had died in childbirth just that February.

Eric Duncan might never have come to America if I hadn't been grieving so much for my daughter Kebeh. Eric's original reason for coming to Dallas in May was to be at Karsiah's graduation, but he also came to comfort me. By the time he had his ticket, it was September: seven months had passed since Kebeh's death, and still I cried all day.

Here is the story of her death that keeps going around and around in my mind. In February 2014, she was thirty-one, pregnant with her fifth child. She went into labor on a Saturday when all the banks in Monrovia were closed. When her husband took her to the hospital, they said there was a problem with the pregnancy. Kebeh was bleeding and needed to have blood, but they had no cash. Her husband went to find friends who might give him the money.

She called me: "Mommy, pray for me. I am bleeding so much! My baby is dead, but I need them to save my life."

She put the nurse on the phone, and I said, "Why can't you help that child? She is bleeding. She is losing her life. Can you give me the doctor?"

"We have to have money first," the nurse said.

"I will send the money," I told her. "You will have it Monday." But they would not operate until they had it.

When the nurse handed the phone back to my daughter, I said to her, "Let's pray to God."

I heard Kebeh begging them to help her, but they wouldn't. I could hear them walking around and talking of other things while my daughter lay dying. I was praying, telling her not to be afraid, but she was so weak that she stopped talking. She made just a little noise, "Eh," and that was all. This daughter was the best of them. Of my five girls, she was the sweetest, and always happy.

"I wasn't there," I told myself. "I should have been there." The guilt inside me is so strong. Maybe if I had been in Monrovia, I would have had the money to pay the doctors. Maybe I would have talked them into helping her.

Even in September, I was so grieving Kebeh that I could not eat or sleep. I had stopped going to work. In my job as a certified nurse assistant caring for old people, I am patient and they all love me. They say I am always happy. But now my sadness was so great that even the Alzheimer's patients could see it. Seeing me so different made them unhappy and they became agitated. I had to lay aside my sadness to comfort and calm them, but these people feel what other people are feeling. They could always feel that my sadness was there.

It was after my daughter's death in February that my relationship with Timothy's father, Peterson, ended. We had not been happy with each other for a long time. And now I was so sad. We parted.

Eric had often called to talk about Karsiah, but after February he also talked to me about my loneliness and grief.

He had loved us all for many years. He remembered when
Kebeh was a girl. He remembered hard things that happened long ago that we don't talk about to others. Such
old friends don't have to say everything because they know
so much already. He told me about what good children my
grandchildren were. Eric described my daughter's house.
She had a good husband, he said. He told me how smart
she was, and people at her job respected her so much.

I was hungry for that talk from such a gentle man. I had
missed so much of my daughter's life. Now there was no
more of it to share. Every minute of my life in America, I
had longed for the children I'd left: such deep yearning
and so many old hopes. They gave my life meaning. They
were the desires I took most often to God.

It seemed I would never stop being sad. So one day Karsiah called his father and told him I could not stop crying.
"You must come and make her happy," Karsiah told Eric.

Eric had said, "Of course I must come. I have been begging your mother to let me come. I have no relationship
and she has no relationship. We should be together. I will
take away her sadness."

Then Karsiah spoke of his father again to me. He said
that only his father could make me well again, and that I
must send for him.

And so I did, and while he waited to come to me, Eric
saw another pregnant girl who needed help. He helped
her. She died. But he didn't tell me. After news of how Eric
helped this girl was on television, some Liberians were saying that Eric was the father of the girl's baby. But my son
who lives in Monrovia checked it out and called to tell me
that it was not true.

So why didn't Eric tell me about helping that girl? I will never know. If I had known, would I have said, "Don't come"?

Maybe, but maybe not. A woman dying in childbirth is not so unusual in Liberia, which has the eighth-highest maternal death rate in the world. Out of 100,000 deliveries, 770 women die in childbirth every year. So maybe this girl's death would not have made me afraid about Eric coming.

I do not think Eric knew he had Ebola. No one in that neighborhood suspected that Marthalene had Ebola. But I am a cautious woman. I might have asked how he was feeling. I might have told him to delay his trip until we could be sure.

We will never know how different the next month might have been if Eric had told me the story of that girl. One thing is for sure: he should have told me.

# CHAPTER SIX

# My Church, My Community

By the time Eric got to Dallas, my four daughters who ended up living in Guinea had gotten visas and had come over on the refugee program in 2005 and 2006. With Eric's nephew Oliver Smallwood living with me and also Jeffrey Cole, a nephew of Kebeh's husband, finally I was not so lonely. My daughters were grown now and lived in apartments near me. They worked in health care like I did.

As Karsiah was making plans to go to college, lots of colleges were scouting him. Then he hurt his shoulder, and he didn't have so many offers. But he still planned on college. He is a determined boy, and he found a place at Angelo State University.

I told my son many times, "If you go to school, you're not going to work hard like me. You see I am working hard. My legs are hurting. I only have thirty minutes to take lunch, and sometimes I can't even take it. I don't have time to take the break. Even dragging because of this arthritis, I still make it to work. You need to go to school. We are just laborers. While we are breaking down and working hard, the people with good education are enjoying their life. They work less and make more. If you want to learn and stay out of trouble, you can become whoever you want to be."

To others we may look like poor people, but we are not hungry anymore. Our children go to school. We have a chance to have a better future. At first when I came to America I was so lonely for Africa where everyone's doors are open and people are always going in and out of each other's houses. In America you have to make an appointment even to visit someone.

But now I have many loved ones here. They come to my house. If I am sad or lonely they stay with me. I make sure I have many beds and one big bed in my bedroom so they can always stay. I cook a lot of food in my big pots and pans, enough for everyone to eat and have more for the next day. My daughters never wake up in the morning thinking that their children will have only one meal that day.

When I came to America, I didn't think about being a citizen. I didn't even know I could; I was just so grateful that America let me come here. I was not even dreaming about more. Then I heard that after five years if you had no bad reputation and if you live under the laws and regulations, you can be a citizen. My thought was that I should prove that I appreciate being in this country.

In 2009, I started studying to become an American citizen. I studied for a month, working through a workbook, listening to a CD. The test had ten questions. I answered all of them right. When the woman giving me the test looked up and said, "Congratulations," I said, "Thank God."

When Eric came, he would see that all the Liberians here know me. My nickname is 214, the area code of my phone number. I can remember anybody's telephone number if they just tell it to me one time. That means that I can always remember to call when people need anything.

Liberians also joke that I am called 1-800 because people from anywhere can call me. Whatever they ask me to do, I do it. If they need something and I have money, I give it to them. Whenever I hear that someone has come from Liberia, I buy something for them, even if it's only something for a dollar, a little gift. Or maybe I cook them some African food.

I take this gift to them and I say, "Welcome to America."

Then I tell them what my father told me: in America you must never overlook your work. God is first. Work is second.

If the new refugee is a woman, I say, "You have to be a strong, brave woman. Even if you're in love with a man, don't depend on him. Be on time for your work. Forget Liberian time. That is not American time. Go to work on time and that way it will be okay."

I keep advising and helping these women, and some of them call me their play mom. I help a lot of people and a lot of people help me.

I have always loved God, but I did not go to church all the time in America. Karsiah was baptized at the Skillman Church of Christ, not too far from where we live. His uncle who was in prison started going there because this church had a ministry for those who had been prisoners. Karsiah went with him, and some people in the church made friends with my son. A couple in the church are his godparents now. They love him and help him very much. In 2011, he went with the church youth group to help fix houses torn up by tornadoes in Joplin, Missouri.

When three of my Liberian nieces came to Dallas two years ago, some people at a Dallas church called Wilshire

Baptist started to help them. They heard about my nieces through a Christian program for immigrants. This church is about five miles from where I live, very nice, with a tall steeple, big buildings, and flowers around it. Maybe not the kind of church people think I would go to. And I would not think so, either, but these people reached out to me so much that I wanted to be with them.

Wilshire Baptist Church has 3,000 members and a $4 million budget to spend every year. Wilshire is not the richest church in Dallas, but compared to my family, its members are rich. Many Wilshire people have been Baptists all their lives. About half are Republicans and half are Democrats, and most are white. They are well-schooled people, the kind of people Karsiah will one day be.

Dallas has lots of Baptist churches. Most are Southern Baptist, and Wilshire was also until the 1990s, when the Southern Baptist Convention stopped focusing on things people at Wilshire think are important, like giving people the freedom to think about the Bible in different ways. After sixty-three years of being a church, Wilshire has paid off all its buildings and made them nice. Now the church is helping poor people with the money that used to be spent on buildings.

Wilshire has a minister whose whole job is helping poor people and helping change things that are unfair in society. When she repeats one popular saying about helping people, she makes it different. She says Wilshire must give people a fish, teach them to fish, and break down the fence that's around the fishing pond.

When Dallas African Americans protested that George Zimmerman, who killed the Florida boy Trayvon Martin, was turned loose by the jury, Wilshire's senior pastor George Mason was the only white minister there. Wilshire is partners with an African American church in Dallas in trying to make payday lenders stop charging so much interest when people borrow money. Wilshire calls them predatory lenders.

It was the Sunday-school class of Wilshire seniors called Open Bible that first found out about my three nieces and decided to help them. One of the Open Bible members is a retired Texas Instruments executive named Max Post, whose wife had died. Max has the nice way of being that sometimes comes when someone has been a Christian all his life. He is a thin, gentle man who will not judge anyone badly and is always wanting to help people who haven't had such good lives.

So Max went to where my nieces were living with their uncle and asked what he could do to help them. He thought their uncle might say that they needed food or clothes, but he didn't say that. The uncle said the thing they needed most was to learn about computers. This was lucky, because Max helps people learn about computers in a class at the church. So he started teaching my nieces. Two other retired people in the Open Bible class—John Coates, who used to be an investigator with the US Office of Special Counsel, and his wife, Mig, who was a teacher's aide—took my nieces out for ice cream and to the YMCA. People in the Open Bible Class helped the youngest, Christina, enroll in high school. They helped the other two, Gbor and Agnes, enroll in community college.

One day after my daughter Kebeh died in February 2014, Max brought Agnes home after classes to my apartment.

Agnes was sleeping at my house because I was so sad. I had two pictures of Kebeh. When I looked at those pictures, I always cried. So I was crying and Max saw. He asked me who the girl was, and I told him it was my Liberian daughter Kebeh who died and that I was not able to attend her memorial service. My sadness went into Max and I could see it on his face.

"We could have a memorial service for your daughter here," he said in his soft way. "We could have it in the church or here in your home. My church will send a pastor."

Maybe such a service would help me get over my grief. "Here would be good," I said. Max arranged for it to happen almost right away. We put chairs in rows in the big sitting room of my apartment and tables to the side with lots of African food. Max came to the memorial service and brought food. John and Mig Coates also came with food. A Liberian pastor prayed, and we all sang godly songs. A young Wilshire pastor with a black beard and glasses named Brent Newberry read from the Scripture and said comforting things. It was his first memorial service as a pastor, and he was so sad to see our grief.

I cried and cried, and so did my daughters. Max, John, and Mig hugged us all and looked as sad as we did. Afterward, we all ate the food. Some of it was too hot for the people from Wilshire. Having this memorial service made me feel not so terrible.

I was so grateful that one Sunday I picked up my nieces and we went to Wilshire to attend Open Bible Sunday-school class. The church was so big that I was lost when I walked in. But my nieces had been before, and they knew where to go, up the elevator and down the hall to a class that had Open Bible written on a card on the door.

Some churches are so nice on the outside, but the people inside are not so nice. At Wilshire both outside and people inside are nice. Max saw me and came to hug me. Then he hugged my nieces. Mig and John came to hug and say how happy they were to see me. Liberians are people who like to touch each other, and I was glad to be in a place where so many people hugged us. That Sunday-school class makes me feel so wanted. When I go there, they all greet me, and they say, "Oh, we are so glad to see you." And I see in their faces that they are glad.

These people make me feel that I am one of them. They welcome us, and they show compassion for the girls and me. They accept us as one in Christ. Every week in our class, we pray for people who are sick or unhappy. I ask them to pray for Liberia.

In church services, my nieces and I always sit on the right hand of the preacher just about halfway up. Sometimes my daughters and my grandchildren come with me. We almost fill up the pew. Wilshire has a big organ with silver pipes, and every week big bouquets of flowers are set in front on both sides of the pulpit. The walls are a light pink that makes the air glow, and white plantation shutters are at the tall windows along the side of the church. Sometimes people bring horns and saxophones and bells to play in the service.

This church is different from Liberian churches. Not so loud. No shouting. The music is different. In Liberian churches, the songs can make you feel like dancing. Not so much at Wilshire. Nobody speaks in tongues. When there are prayers, nobody raises their hands up to God. Nobody shouts "Amen" from the congregation. I love Liberian churches. But Wilshire is where God told me to be.

The main Wilshire pastor is named George Mason. He is a big man, more than six feet tall, who must bend down to hug me. Everyone calls him George. I call him Pastor George because to use just the first name of God's anointed one is not to be so respectful.

On Sundays in the pocket of his jacket Pastor George wears a folded handkerchief that matches his shirt or his tie. He loves to golf, and once he said in a sermon that he is a country club Christian. People always remember to say that Pastor George was a quarterback at the University of Florida. He still loves football, but he does not talk much about it in his sermons.

"That would be pandering," he says, because in Texas football is so popular. People hardly ever mention that he has a PhD. He is a brainy preacher who quotes poets and philosophers but always preaches from the Bible. Other preachers tease him about being too handsome. These things give Pastor George some glamour. But people at Wilshire don't mention Pastor George's looks much. They see him in all the ways he is good, not just looking so.

He is from New York, the son and grandson of harbor pilots, an East Coast Baptist, he says, the kind who comes from east of the Mississippi and thinks about being Baptist in ways that go back to early days of America when Baptists were fighting for freedom and defending people nobody listened to. I love these ideas so much. They are the ideas that so many people in Africa love about America.

Many people come to Wilshire because of Pastor George's preaching. But then they say, "He is a good preacher, but if you really want to see him at his best, you have to see him when he's being a pastor." They mean that he cares for people, not just preaching about caring. He is known for opening his arms wide and pulling people to him.

Every week he talks about how Christians should help each other and be brothers and sisters to one another. We are practicing for how it will be in heaven, he says. We must try to be like Jesus, and if we try, God will help us.

Some Sundays, new parents bring a baby to the front of the church. The family stands behind the baby: grandparents, aunts, uncles, and cousins. Pastor George puts a diaper on the shoulder of his nice suit and takes the baby. He tells the parents that they have been given this baby by God, but that the baby is not just theirs, but also God's.

Then he walks around the church, talking to the baby so that everyone else can hear. He welcomes the baby. When he gets back to the front, he asks everyone if they will love and protect the baby and help the child through life. And everyone in the church says, "We will."

My niece Agnes is pregnant now and when her baby comes, Pastor George will bless it while we all stand in front of the church. This blessing is part of what he calls extending the canopy of grace. Before the service ends, Pastor George says that anyone who wants to come forward can join the church. Anyone who hasn't been baptized can be baptized.

In Africa, I was in Jehovah's Witnesses from birth, like my brother who was killed by the soldiers because he would not fight. But Witnesses are so strict. When I was younger, I was maybe a little bit of a bad girl. I couldn't be a Witness. All my life I have loved God so much. I read my Bible and I pray. I trust God.

But I have never been baptized. So one Sunday when Pastor George said, "Come up if you want to join the church,"

I heard God telling me that I should. I thought, *This is the place God wants me to be.*

Wilshire has some African Americans, not many. And I don't think there are any Liberians in the church except for my family and friends. But I didn't even think about this church being full of white people because this is where we are all God's children.

So when I went to the front and Pastor George said, "Would you like to be baptized?" I said I would.

Then he said to the people, "If you will welcome Louise and promise to love and support her as our sister in Christ, will you say, 'Thanks be to God'?"

Everyone said, "Thanks be to God." Then a long line of people stood to shake my hand and tell me how happy they were to have me there.

In June, three months before Eric arrived, I was baptized in the Baptist way, under water. A little pool of water is built into the wall behind the choir where baptisms take place. One of the lady ministers, Tiffany Wright, held my back and my face and tilted me back into the water until my head went under. Because I was nervous, I was talking a lot. She looked nervous, too. When we went into the water she tilted me back, but my nose was still sticking out of the water.

She pushed me more until my whole face was under. She said, "I baptize you in the name of the Father, the Son, and the Holy Spirit." As she lifted me from the water, dripping, I walked away, praising God in my spirit.

Since that great day, terrible things have happened. My actions brought Eric to America using a ticket I bought with borrowed money. Reaching for love, I brought tragedy. The father of my son and the love of my life died a terrible death, alone. Friends turned against me. Strangers wished for me dead. I was outcast, under guard, my children in danger.

But God watched to help me. It was God giving me the privilege to be an American citizen. It was God guiding me to join Wilshire. I am a citizen who does no wrong. I obey the laws. I love America and God. This is why citizens of this nation and people of the church came to help me in my sorrow.

# CHAPTER SEVEN

# My Spirit Took Him In

By the time Eric arrived, I had a job that helped me help others. I had many of my children with me in America. I had my God; but something was still missing. Having Eric around made me think I could have more. I still grieved my daughter, but having a man with me who called her "daughter" and grieved with me helped so much.

When Eric kissed me for the first time in Texas, I turned my head so he was kissing me on the cheek, not the mouth.

"Hello, Mrs. Duncan," he said.

"You are missing the mark there," I said. "I am not Mrs. Duncan yet. I have not changed my name. I am Louise Troh."

"You are always Mrs. Duncan to me, and we will make it even truer."

Then he said, "Oh, sweetheart, many, many years I tried so hard, and finally I came to America through you. I am so grateful to God for bringing me to you. If I was a woman I would cry, but I am a man, so I won't. I can't believe it. Miracles happen."

We had always been talking about how we would marry, but now he started talking about something more—an oath. "From now on, till death will do us part," he said. "I'm not going to let you go and we are not going to be parted. When we are married that won't be enough. We are going to go and take an oath. To the end of this life, we are going to be together. We are brother and sister."

As I listened to Eric talk, it felt just like before. From the very beginning he had fastened onto me, refusing to be discouraged. He was talking like he had twenty years ago during those months when he came every day to talk me into giving him a chance. We were beginning again as if we never parted. He hadn't been with me for much more than an hour and already my fears were going away.

Eric had been riding on the plane so long. No bath for two days. I started running water for him. The tub was filling up so I took him to the closet that held Karsiah's clothes.

"These are your son's clothes," I said, pulling out T-shirts and some pants. "What do you want to wear?"

He held a T-shirt up to him, and then picked a pair of khaki pants. "Are these my son's clothes?" he asked. "Is he this big?"

"Yes. When you see your son, you will be looking up when you talk to him."

He stood there for a long time with his hands in his pockets. He looked like he was about to cry. Then he said, "I will wear these clothes, and I will feel the spirit of my son. I will feel close to him."

After he cleaned himself, I cooked some food for him. I made him potato leaf soup, my favorite. He wasn't very hungry.

I said, "I don't cook so good."

"You do. Tell people that your husband likes your food." He had always been that way, trying to make me feel better.

If he had to say something, he would not say it right away—just think so that he could say it the best way.

My son Timothy had been at a football game. When he came in, he was frowning, looking at Eric without much friendliness. But Eric opened his arms to him and said, "I am so happy to meet you, Timothy. I am going to love you like my own son. When I get a job, we will go many places together."

Timothy smiled at him then.

The boys were watching TV while we ate at the table. Timothy went to spend the night with his cousin. My three granddaughters—Grace, seven; Rose, six; and Knowledge, five—came to spend the night. They would sleep on the mattresses.

After Eric finished eating, I said to them, "Well, guys, we need to get some rest."

When we went to my bedroom, I said, "Sleep here so I can monitor you for a few days. Then we can join together."

He said, "Do you have somebody?"

"No. I wouldn't have had you come here if I had somebody," I said.

"I have been saving myself for you," he said, looking at me so tenderly. "I am a changed man. I've been baptized. I want to live a good life with you."

But he also knew that I was thinking that he had come from a country that has the virus. I was thinking about Ebola. I didn't worry that he would bring it from Monrovia when we were talking before he came. I hadn't thought about that as a danger. But I am a cautious woman. I work in health care. Maybe I just needed that reassurance.

Thousands of people had already died in Liberia from Ebola. We knew that a person would not be infected and contagious unless their temperature rose high. Waiting a few days couldn't make so much difference after being apart for so long.

But Eric said, "You don't need to worry about that. I don't have anything. They monitored me so much at the airport. You won't even believe how much they screened me. There is no danger. If I was sick with Ebola, they would have never let me out of Liberia."

And so I was convinced. I believed completely that he was healthy, and so did he. Looking back it may seem odd, but I never thought about Ebola again until the hospital told me they were going to test Eric for it. When he told me about the airport screening, I accepted that he was not infected. Through all the illness to come I thought other things might be wrong, but not Ebola.

We had both waited for each other for a long time. We were mature people who had not been with anyone else for a long time. We made love that night without using protection and fell asleep in each other's arms. I woke up after a while and pulled away from him. I was not accustomed to sleeping with anyone.

He woke up and said, "Why are you moving away from me? I want you to be right by my side always."

I said, "No. I don't want to sleep with a man's arm around me. I must sleep a little way away from you." That's how we slept, but when we woke up we were together again.

At 4:00 a.m. Sunday morning, we woke up with a telephone call from his mother in North Carolina, so happy that Eric was finally in América. She couldn't stop calling to say how happy she was that we were together.

Eric handed me his phone, and he said, "That's your mother-in-law. She has always loved you so much and you loved her." It's true that she always loved me, from that first day when she saw me dancing, and she said to her daughters, "I wish that girl would be one of my son's girlfriends."

Later she told me, "My spirit took you in. My son and I are in love with you. God picked you." If Eric had different girlfriends, she wouldn't even be interested in them. And I was not interested in other men once I met Eric. It was the same with him and me as it had been with his mother and me. It didn't happen right away because I wasn't looking for a man, but as we were together more, my spirit took him in and never let him go.

In Dallas that Sunday morning Eric and I stayed in the bed talking about the life we were going to have.

"What you have done for me, you don't even know," he said. "I will never try to hurt you. If I should ever make a mistake, bring me into this room and tell me. Don't let anyone in my family know. Just bring me into the room, and if I know I have done anything wrong, I am not so big that I can't say I am sorry."

He was still saying that we must get married right away.

"I don't have money for marriage," I told him. We would go to the courthouse and that cost money. Later I wanted to be married at Wilshire Baptist Church, but first the courthouse. I told him maybe we could marry in October.

I have a friend in town and one in Philadelphia that I called about the marriage. Before Eric came I told them, "You need to send some contribution." One said she would send me $150 and the other would send $150. I needed about $500 and could supply the rest.

I had to work that Sunday so I could not go to church. Eric wanted to go to church with me. I told him how very nice the people at Wilshire were to me. But first he very much wanted to go to Skillman Church of Christ to meet his son's godparents and thank them for helping Karsiah. He was feeling good, but still so tired. My daughter Youngor told him that he shouldn't go to church. He might not be as friendly and remember the things he wanted to say when he met so many new people. She said he should just stay at home and rest.

I cooked some food that Eric liked, some catfish in palm oil and some greens. He didn't like meat, except for sausage. I cooked a lot so anyone who came in could have some. A few people started coming by, family and my friends who all wanted to meet Eric. They knew he was my longtime love. Some of them knew him from Liberia or from the Ivory Coast. My nieces came to say hello. He called his nephew's girlfriend in North Carolina that morning, and they started singing a godly song.

Eric had not been so much a Christian when we were together, but he had changed. He had been baptized and he loved church. So she was helping him have church right there in my apartment. He stood up and spread his arms and sang that song so loud and good. I never knew he could sing. And he was dancing around the room a little, so happy.

Then I got ready to go to work. I went into the bathroom to take a shower. He wanted to go in with me. I said, "No, you don't need to go in there."

He said, "I want to be everywhere you are, Mrs. Duncan."

I laughed when he called me that. "You are just like your mother, always wanting to be with me and to touch me," I said.

His age had changed, but nothing else. He was a real man now with gray hair in his beard. "Wow," I said. "Fifteen years have gone by. We are older people now."

"You look just the same to me," he said. Eric was always optimistic, always looking for the good things in a situation. It is true that I was older and I knew he must see that. But I am not as skinny and sad as I was in Africa. My skin is not so dry, and I am not as ugly as I was in those hard times.

He called his father in Africa that day to let him know that he was in Dallas. "Be patient," he told his father. "I am going to get a job and send you money."

After I got ready for work, he walked me to the car and kissed me. I told him, "Don't kiss me on the mouth. If you do that, I will embarrass you by turning away." So he always hugged me, holding me to show how much he loved me, and kissing my cheek. But also on my mouth and I didn't embarrass him.

When I came home, he was sitting near the window watching for my car, and he came out into the parking lot to meet me and walk me inside. Almost every day of our time together, he walked me to the car when I left for work and waited for me outside to walk me in when I came home.

I got home around 3:30 p.m. I asked him if he'd eaten and he said, "No, sweetheart. I have waited on you."

"You should eat something," I said. "Even if you just eat some fruit." But he liked to eat with me. I would cook the African food that we like, fresh food, not canned. Eric loved fish the best. So he would tell me to cook fish with soup. He loved catfish in palm butter. Secondly he loved sausage. He would say, "Cook me a little sausage." He didn't like spicy food because he had an ulcer in his stomach.

Monday was September 22, our son's nineteenth birthday. Eric called our Karsiah very early in the morning so that he could be the first to wish him a happy birthday. Karsiah was at school at Angelo State University, 270 miles away. He did not have a car to travel, and he had to study. He spent all his time practicing football or studying. It was his first semester, and he wanted very much to have good grades. So he studied for hours every day. He planned to see his father when he came home at Thanksgiving.

"Wake up and talk to our son," Eric said. "Don't you know that we have a nineteen-year-old son today?"

Eric said he could not wait until Thanksgiving to see his son. He wanted to go to the college on Wednesday. I told him that I would take him the next week when I was on vacation. I laughed at seeing him so happy. But we would not make that trip. By the Wednesday we were to visit Karsiah, Eric Duncan would be world-famous in a way that nobody wanted.

While I was getting ready for work, Eric would wake Timothy so that he would not be late for school. After Timothy got ready, Eric would walk with him part of the way to school. Timothy was still wondering about this new man in my life. I told him that after Uncle Eric got a job, he would be taking him places and buying him things—maybe to the mall for shoes. Timothy loves athletic shoes. He wants shoes from Macy's, the best shoes, not from Payless. When I told him Eric would buy him shoes, my son was happy.

Eric slept in the same bed with me every night. It's a king-size bed, and he slept by the wall. In the night, we'd be talking in the bed and sometimes Eric would snore. I would hit him and he would say, "Oh, I am sorry."

I said, "Why are you sleeping so much?"

"It's because I had that long ride on the plane," he said.

When I would go to bed, he would always come to lie next to me with his arms around me and his hands stroking my skin. I am not used to so much closeness.

"Why can't you leave a person's skin alone?" I would ask.

"It is a package," he would say. "You and I are together. So you have to deal with me for the rest of your life."

Often we talked of my late daughter, Kebeh. Other people had cried with me. They had tried to comfort me. But it was Eric who knew what I most needed to hear—that her life had been happy. He told me many people loved my daughter and so many came to her funeral.

"You would not believe the nice cars they had," he said. "And she looked so good. Not like she was dead—just asleep. It was like the funeral of a queen."

He told me what a good husband she had. Her husband had blamed himself for not having taken money from the bank before the weekend. He said he should have hidden it and had it ready so that he could pay the hospital when she was ready to deliver the baby. But my daughter had borne four children. No one thought the fifth baby would be so hard. No one thought that the hospital would refuse to help her. Liberian women didn't always die so much in childbirth. Now the hospitals are so bad and women die.

On Tuesday morning, Eric was still so tired and now a little bit dizzy. I thought he was just still recovering from travel. It takes some time to get used to the time change. It might have been Tuesday night that I told him about the abortion. He didn't know that I had been pregnant with his baby, of course.

"Why did you never tell me?" he asked.

"There was nothing you could do. I could not keep that baby. And why would I tell you such a thing on the phone? You were too far away. I had to work to survive."

Then he said, "Sweetheart, we have to have one American baby to replace that one we lost. It's not too late for us. We will have our baby and be a family."

I laughed at that idea. "I am too old to have babies."

"I am serious about this," he said.

"You better erase this from your mind," I said. "Karsiah is our son. He will give **us** grandbabies. They will be our babies."

We talked all the time about how we would marry. Every time, he would start talking about us taking the oath. "I want us to take an oath that we will always be together. Husband and wife until death parts us. Not only husband and wife but also sister and brother."

I didn't know why he wanted the oath, but I said that I would take it. After his death I thought, "Did he know that he was going to die?"

"Why are you so particular about this oath?" I asked.

He said, "I want to prove to you that I am yours and you are mine forever."

"Come on, boy, stop lying to me," I would say. Because maybe I was still a little afraid. When we were in Ivory Coast, he was such a cheater. He loved to run.

"I'm not playing with this," he said, not smiling at all. "I am telling you the truth."

Eric was never angry or complaining. Even when he was a young man, he never raised his voice. When he got really mad, you could only tell because his eyes would turn red. But if you asked him what was wrong, he would say, "Oh, nothing." Then he would be over it, and he would do whatever I told him. He hadn't changed at all.

One of the first things I told Eric was that he would have to keep the bathroom clean. I always spray the toilet with disinfectant before and after I use it. If other people don't spray the toilet, I go in, put on my gloves, and do it for them. I also make sure people wash their hands. I have regular soap and antibacterial soap for them to use. So I told Eric and he agreed.

When he would go to the bathroom, I would listen for the water running. If I didn't hear it, I would say, "Did you wash your hands?"

If he said, "Yes, I did," but I did not hear water, I would say, "No, sweetheart, you did not."

And he would go back and wash his hands. I'm picky that way. All my children know it. Working in a nursing home where everything has to be clean, I learned these ways. I am always washing my hands.

Eric was tired but not feeling sick when he first came, but as Tuesday went on, he began to feel worse. When he called his brother Wilfred, in Arizona, he told him that he was feeling bad. His brother said, "Jet lag. Welcome to America." They laughed.

"You wouldn't believe all the people she has brought here to America. I can't even imagine how many," he told his brother. It was true that I created a good life. He even liked that big room with too many chairs. "It still looks pretty," he said.

I didn't have to tell him why there were three mattresses. "Too many grandbabies," he said. "You love them so much. If someone cries because they don't want to share, you give them their own mattress."

He couldn't believe how much stuff I had. "You have so many bedsheets, towels, dishes. All these comforters. I can't believe all this. I love your life. You make yourself happy."

"Yes," I said. "I feel good."

He had brought from Africa a lot of music, 250 songs to play on a computer. "We will have lots of music," he said.

"And we will dance. When I am well, we will always be listening to music and dancing."

On Tuesday during the day, he didn't show that he was sick, but that night he started having a headache and some fever.

A few of my friends and family were coming by, just to say hello. They would run in and meet him, not usually staying long because everyone is working. Sometimes Eric would be lying on a mattress in the sitting room. He would get up and say hello and usually hug them because he thought of my family as his family, and my friends as his friends.

On Wednesday Eric's fever showed more. I first noticed it when I was hugging him.

"Your skin is hot," I said. "You must take some medicine."

He would take some Tylenol and sweat. In a little while he would say, "I feel better."

But after two hours, he would start running a fever again. I said, "Keep swallowing the pills." Every time he did, the fever went down.

My daughter Youngor's two-year-old son, Prophet, loved Eric right away. Prophet knew Eric felt bad. By Wednesday, Eric was saying that his stomach hurt, so Prophet would put his hands on Eric's stomach and pray for him. He did this five or six times, crawling up in Eric's lap and looking up into Eric's face, already loving him so much. Later, when Eric was in the hospital and his picture was everywhere on the TV, Prophet would see his face and go to the television to touch it, saying, "Eric."

That Wednesday I noticed that Eric was talking a little different. He would have some plan or idea that he wanted us to think about, but he would add, "After I get well." That was the only way I knew how bad he felt.

I have known some other people who come from Africa with a little fever. After a while it goes away. But they might feel a little bad for two weeks or more. I even knew one woman who went to the hospital and stayed two weeks before she was well. I wasn't alarmed. I thought, *Eric has some minor problem and will get better.*

When I told him about these people who had been sick and gotten well, he said, "That's probably it." At the airport they took his temperature many times. They questioned him many times. There was no Ebola in his neighborhood before he came. And his fever went down with only Tylenol. I did not think Tylenol would take care of something as terrible as fever caused by Ebola.

So I did not suspect. Did I suspect a little, deep within myself? No, I did not.

Once again on Wednesday when I came in from work, he hadn't eaten.

"I bought you some fruit. You must eat," I said. I thought maybe not eating was part of his problem—and maybe not drinking enough water. I kept telling him to drink more water, but he didn't like water. Wednesday night was the first night we did not make love.

On Thursday afternoon I drove home from work expecting Eric would be getting better. He'd been in the country since Sunday, long enough for his sleep to be getting better and for him to be getting adjusted to the difference in water. Eric wasn't having diarrhea or vomiting, just some fever, and that wasn't too high, maybe a little over 100°. It all seemed minor, the kind of little sickness people have all the time, especially after a long journey.

# CHAPTER EIGHT

## *Fever*

By now it was the end of Eric's fourth full day in America. I always left my cell phone with him, so I did not talk to him after I left home at 6:30 a.m. Getting up and out so early is hard, but I am never late. If my card says that I punched in a few minutes late, I don't get the full hour of work. So I am on time.

People at the nursing home tease, "Mama Lou really loves that money. She makes sure she gets it all."

Boy, is it a hard job. It can break people down. Lift with the knees and the back, or you can be hurt badly. I have arthritis in my leg because of this lifting. Sometimes I am limping so much that I don't even want people to see me.

Even the residents I help can see how hard my job is. I remember a woman who was so sweet. I was taking care of her and she said, "Louise, I wouldn't take your job for a million dollars. It's dangerous. It's annoying. It's nasty. It's a killing job. I don't know why you chose to do this work."

"Don't discourage me in my job," I said.

"I'm just telling the facts," she said. "Is this what you came from Africa to do?"

"Can we just flip it and talk about something else?" I said. I have to keep a good attitude.

When I am doing something good for other people, I feel good about it. Not everybody understands how to treat the residents. I tell the new employees, "They don't like people to scream at them. If they see that frown on your face, that's going to make them agitated. So just smile and laugh."

One of the residents said, "I love everyone here, but Louise is the best. If Louise tells me to do anything, I will obey." But she always calls me even when I tell her not to call me because I'm going downstairs. She just wants me to be with her. She will call and call, and when I come, I tell her not to call again.

But she says, "I just have to see you."

The nurses are always calling me to help them, too. I tell them to call someone else. But they say, "When we call you, we see that fire in your eyes, and we know that you will do it."

One old lady sits at the front by the door, saying, "Help me. Help me. I need some juice." So when I come in, I don't even put my purse down, just run and grab her some juice. She likes to have a napkin on her head. So when I give her the juice, I put a napkin on her head and she says, "Oh thank you, Miss Louise."

One of them would never take a shower for anyone but me. Her relatives said, "Louise, how do you manage?"

I said, "You just have to be very patient with her." When I go to get her for a shower, she might grab her hairbrush like she is going to hit me, and I laugh, "Hee, hee. You are going to hit me? Please, I just came here to help you. Please don't hurt me. Just go into the bathroom."

When she goes in, she will say, "Shut the door."

I shut the door and repeat, "Okay, okay," in a soft voice, never in a hurry.

Everybody there loves me. I love them. They are part of my family. When I am gone they will call and check on me. "We miss you. We need you back. When are you coming?" I miss them, too, especially those funny residents.

The phone starts ringing every day when I get off: my daughters, my friends, my nieces. So many people are calling me all the time. I have built a good life full of people. We all care for each other. I no longer feel the loneliness of American life. I have imported many of my life's important people from Africa and I have added others. Sometimes I get home at 3:15 p.m. and a carful of people will be waiting for me.

"What took you so long?" they say, like I am a bird flying home and went too slow. "Do you have anything to eat?" Most often I do.

I was looking for Eric in the parking lot that day. It was nice to have him waiting for me. To have Eric greet me with his big smile, kiss me, and walk into the apartment was my day's best part. I am taking care of someone always and now Eric was taking care of me. This life we waited for so long was finally started.

But on that Thursday, September 25, he wasn't in the parking lot. This made me a little worried. I hoped maybe he was sleeping and just hadn't noticed the time.

Then I saw him standing at the top of the stairs outside my apartment. In September, Dallas can be still hot. People are still wearing sandals. But Eric was wearing Karsiah's T-shirt and Timothy's jacket. Timothy likes to wear his things big, so his jacket fit Eric. Two weeks before Eric came, his mother was visiting me and also wore this same jacket. Eric and his mother were alike in many ways. Loving me. Wanting always to be with me—and liking the same clothes. I was laughing a little at Eric liking that same jacket, but his first words made me stop thinking happy thoughts.

"I need to go to the hospital," he said. Eric had a nice deep, strong voice, but it wasn't strong that day.

"What did you say?" I asked him as I climbed the stairs. I slipped out of my shoes at the door. I always leave those shoes at the door. Nursing homes have a lot of germs and viruses. You don't know what you're getting on you. So I leave my work shoes outside.

"I said I need to go to the hospital."

It was afternoon. Timothy would be getting off from school soon. He would be going to sports practice. The other children might also be coming over. Then heavy rush-hour traffic would start, and it would be hard to get through the traffic. I don't like to drive in traffic.

"Do you want to wait and go to the hospital tomorrow?" I asked.

He said, "No, I need to go now."

He waited for me to go inside, and then he followed me. I was worried about him. Liberians are tough. We don't go to the doctor for every little thing. When we get a cold or the flu, we make a hot hot-pepper drink that makes our eyes start to water and our nose run. Our whole body is burning up from that pepper drink. Then we feel better, no more fever, no running nose. The cold is gone—even flu. To go to the hospital would be big. I was not aware that he was so sick.

As soon as Eric got into the apartment, he sat down. His head drooped and his face sagged.

"I am so cold. And I am so weak. I can't even pick up my head. I feel dizzy. My head hurts and my stomach hurts so much."

"Let me take a shower and change my clothes," I said. "Then I will take you."

I always shower as soon as I come home. I wear scrubs to work. I like having a uniform, but I take it off and put it in a special bag. I don't mix it with my other clothes. I wash my uniform in hot water for safety. That day I took a bath and then changed into other clothes, blue jeans with a blue T-shirt.

When I came out of the bedroom with clean clothes on, Eric was lying on a mattress. The big television was on; it almost always is. He'd fallen asleep all curled up around his stomach like a child. The best thing for him would be to rest. I put another blanket on him.

Then I went into the kitchen to make us some food. When I came from work I'd asked him if he had eaten. He said, "No, would you please make me some soup?"

Eric's way of asking for anything was always gentle so that you wanted to help him. He was grateful for everything. Even in the last days of his life, he was the same.

I made pepper soup and put it in a glass.

He said, "Please, you know I don't like hot things." He meant temperature hot *and* spicy hot. He didn't like either one.

I put a little spice in it: "That will be good for your fever," I said. He waited until it was lukewarm.

"Drink it all," I said.

He did. He started to sweat on his face, and I said, "See, that's helping your fever."

Timothy came in around 6:00 p.m. because he practices football every day. Oliver came in from work around 9:00 p.m. Jeffrey was home, and I gave them all food.

"Here, you need to have water," I said, giving Eric water in one of the big red plastic Solo cups I always use. With so many children around, I don't like to use glasses that might break. With these cups, everything is clean and there is no washing.

"I don't want to drink. I am cold," he said.

"Then you have to drink warm water."

"I don't like water."

"You have to drink to keep yourself hydrated. The fever can make your body lose too much water, and then you will be in trouble." I know how important this is from being around old people. So I did not stop telling him. He would drink, but only when I was there to make him do it.

He'd slept and eaten and drunk warm water, but he still looked bad. His skin looked good when he arrived. Now the color was ashy—not so good.

"Do you still want to go to the hospital?" I asked him.

"Yes. Let's go," he said.

It was dark. I was tired, but waiting another night wouldn't be a good idea. "We can go."

He nodded and slowly got to his feet. I gathered up my keys and purse. Presbyterian Hospital is only about five minutes away. I knew this hospital well. I'd had Timothy at Presbyterian Hospital.

I don't completely trust hospitals. When my daughter Youngor's youngest child, Prophet, was five months old, he got sick, and we took him to Presbyterian Hospital. Then we took him to Medical City, and from there they transferred him to Children's Hospital. The doctors said he needed a liver transplant, but I was afraid of that.

I said, "If you take out his liver, will we get to see it?"

They said no.

"If you give him a new liver, will we get to see it first?"

They said no. But if Prophet didn't get a new liver, they said he would die in a few days.

I said, "God will save this child. He will not die."

We were very afraid, and the doctors said we would be sorry. But one of the doctors said, "If you don't want to do this, don't. He can live for two weeks. So you shouldn't be in a rush. This is a big decision for your family."

I said, "Thank you, these people are all rushing us. Maybe they want to experiment on this boy's liver."

This may sound like I was having crazy thoughts, but to an African it doesn't sound so crazy. Africa has been used to test experimental drugs without anybody being told that they are being used in the test. African Americans have also been used in experiments in this country. I do not like to think that people would do such bad things. But I know that they are done.

So we waited. The doctors said Prophet would start to bleed at the rectum and eyes. After two days, his lips were very dry and started to bleed. Youngor said, "Oh, no, he's going to die."

But I said, "No. His lips are just dry. We will put something on them." The bleeding stopped.

He didn't die in two weeks. He was still sick, but what the doctors said would happen did not. So I said, "Okay. We won't do the transplant."

Youngor and her husband agreed that we wouldn't. Some of the doctors said to Youngor, "Why do you let your mother speak for you?"

And Youngor said, "In African culture, our parents can decide for us. So whatever her decision is, we are going to go by that."

People everywhere started praying for us. But many people thought we were doing the wrong thing. Liberians in the community said, "Wow, we are worried. She took the child home and they might jail her. How can she be strong enough to take that baby home?"

People would call me every day and say, "How is that boy?

Prophet was sick for a year. He would get sick with a fever. Then the fever would go away. We kept praying and praying, and God brought him through.

The doctors said he would not sit, crawl, or walk. But one day Prophet sat up. Then another day, he started dragging himself on the floor after the other kids. I said, "Oh God, you are so amazing."

Later he started crawling on his knees. One day Prophet held the table and he was smiling and I said, "Okay, Prophet, do it, boy, do it."

He started letting go and falling on his bottom and getting up. Then one day, he came to my house and started walking, stomp, stomp, stomp. He's a big boy now, talking trash, two years old, almost three, and well. His father said he is just waiting for his son to get older, and then he will make a surprise visit to those physicians.

Even if I don't trust everything doctors say, I still thought Presbyterian was a good hospital. So I didn't think about taking Eric anywhere else. He was weak and dizzy, but he could walk fine. I pulled into the emergency room parking lot and parked. We walked together into the emergency room doors a few minutes after 10:00 p.m.

Only a few people were sitting there. We went to the desk where the nurse takes your information and then tells you to go sit down and they will call you. No one was standing at the desk, so the nurse helped us right away. She asked for Eric's Social Security number, and I told her that he didn't have one. He had just come from Liberia.

I said, "Liberia in Africa."

Later, the hospital said that Eric told them he came from Africa. I told them even before they asked where he was from. I always said "Liberia." We do not say that we come from Africa; we say the country in Africa.

We had no reason to lie to the hospital. I brought them a sick man. He wanted to get well. We did not think he had Ebola. We know very well the symptoms of Ebola. He wasn't vomiting. He didn't have diarrhea. He was not bleeding from the nose and eyes. If he had those symptoms, we would have told them. I would have been afraid.

For some Americans, Ebola is something far away that's not quite real. But for Liberians in America, it's not so far away. It's a terrible disease that is striking people we know and love. We would never want to bring this disease to America. I love this country. I am a citizen. I would always protect America.

I know how bad Ebola is. I talk to people from Liberia every day. No one there touches when they meet each other, which is something they always used to do. No one even shakes hands. People watch their bodies and monitor

how they feel all the time. They can have their temperatures taken many places. People try not to go into crowds.

I remember when I sent money to my son who lives in
Liberia. When he went to Western Union and the line was
so long, he poured alcohol on himself and all around, and
then asked the crowd, "Why are we all together when we
aren't supposed to be?"

Everyone laughed: "When there's money, we are not
afraid."

In August, all of one large neighborhood in Monrovia
called West Point was quarantined because of Ebola. They
had guards around this neighborhood so that people could
not leave. People inside were so afraid and rioted. If you
didn't have Ebola, you knew that you would get it if you
stayed. Some people were killed trying to escape from the
neighborhood.

People in Liberia who go to the hospital with any kind of
sickness are likely to be sent to the Ebola ward. When one
of my Liberian sons had a fever and diarrhea, he got some
fruit and lots of water, and he stayed away from his family.
He shut himself up in a room to see if he would get well.
If he had gone to a hospital, they would have put him in
the Ebola ward and he would have gotten Ebola. He didn't
want to infect anyone if he had Ebola.

So he stayed in that room until all his symptoms went
away, and he knew that he was well. Maybe this story about
my son was part of the reason that I did not suspect Eric of
having Ebola even when he got so much sicker. We know
that people who come from Africa die of many things.

If Eric had Ebola, we would have wanted the hospital
to know. We would have believed that treatment would

help. When those two American doctors who had Ebola were flown back from Africa, they were very sick, but Western medicine cured them. We believed in the power of US medicine. We trusted the doctors.

I didn't trust the doctors when they wanted to take my grandson's liver out, but whatever was wrong with Eric didn't seem to be so serious. When doctors say they want to do something like replace a child's liver, anyone would question it. But when doctors say that sickness is only minor, everybody is relieved and happy to believe. It was the same with me.

I would not have wanted to take Eric home to my apartment if he had Ebola. I would have wanted him to get treatment right away, to get well and not to infect my family. We went to the hospital for help. We did not go to the hospital to hide anything.

When the admitting nurse told us to wait for a room, we sat on a long couch. I made Eric lie down and put his head on my lap.

"Why are they so slow?" he asked.

"It's not like a real emergency where they bring you in the ambulance. It's not like in Africa where they take care of you fast. Only time they wait on you fast here is when you come in the ambulance," I told him.

In the emergency room, you sit and sit. I think we sat for forty-five minutes. Then they took us to a room right behind the front desk, and a nurse took Eric's vital signs. His temperature was 100.1°—not so high.

The nurse asked Eric to rate his pain on a scale of one to ten, with ten being the highest pain. He said his pain was eight. I knew he was in pain so I was not too surprised.

I could see the pain in his eyes. They were red and held the hurt that eyes have when a person is in pain. But pain did not mean it had to be Ebola. Pain comes with many illnesses.

Then they sent us back to sit again while they looked for a room. After they found a room, they called Eric's name. They asked him to take his shirt off and get in a hospital gown and lie down there. He was complaining about being cold. He had a sheet. But he said, "I'm very, very cold."

"There's nothing we can do," I said. He wanted to wear his clothes but I said, "You can't."

Africans like to be warm. I had been glad that Eric came before the winter so that he wouldn't be cold right away, but I had not thought about how cold the air-conditioning is in Dallas. Buildings can be so cold inside that people bring sweaters to wear when the heat outside is over 100°. In the next few weeks, I would often think about Eric being cold and no one giving him a blanket. In the days to come, I would be even more helpless to stop his suffering.

After about an hour, a doctor came by to check on Eric. He asked if Eric had been around any sick people. Eric said no. No one at my house was sick, and if Eric thought about the pregnant girl he helped in Liberia, he would have been thinking that she died from childbirth, not any kind of illness.

When a nurse came in to ask more questions, I told her that Eric had just come from a long trip, from Liberia. People say that we told them "Africa," but I know that I did not. The nurse and Eric talked about how hard it was to be on such long airplane flights.

So now I had told two nurses that Eric was from Liberia. Why did neither of them think about Ebola? The Liberian

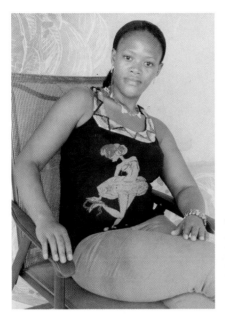

The last photo taken of Louise Troh's late daughter, Kebeh Jallah, in Monrovia, Liberia. (Courtesy of the author)

September 20, 2014: Louise Troh's daughter Nopie Dopoe with Thomas Eric Duncan on the day of his arrival at Dallas–Fort Worth International Airport. (Courtesy of the author)

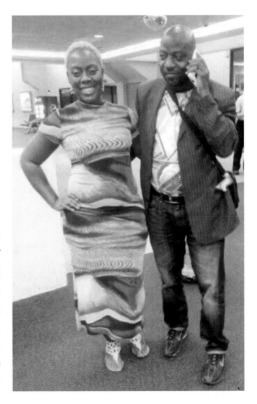

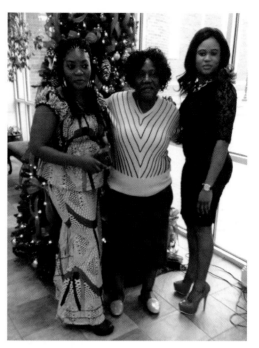

Louise Troh (center), her daughters Youngor Jallah (left) and Mawhen Jallah at Wilshire Baptist Church. (Courtesy of the author)

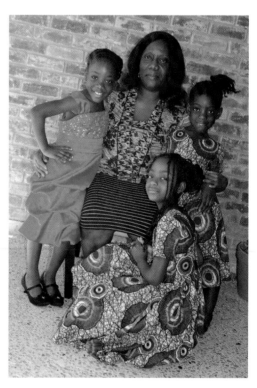

Louise Troh with her granddaughters (from left) Rose, Grace, and Knowledge. (Photo by Jeffrey Cole)

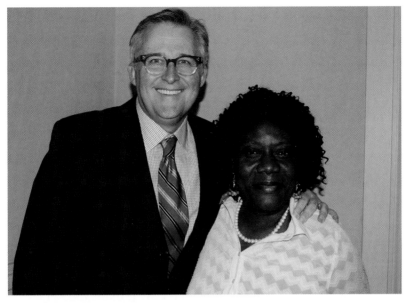

Dallas Wilshire Baptist Church senior pastor George Mason and Louise Troh. (Courtesy of the author)

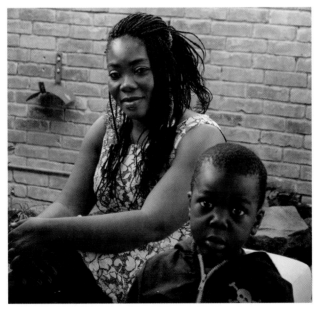

Youngor Jallah, Louise Troh's oldest daughter, with her son Prophet. (Courtesy of the author)

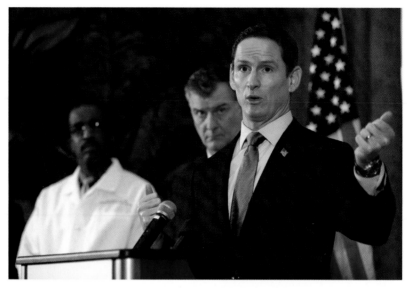

October 1, 2014: Dallas County judge Clay Jenkins answers questions at a press conference about the recent Ebola patient being treated at Texas Health Presbyterian Hospital Dallas. (Photo by Vernon Bryant, *Dallas Morning News*)

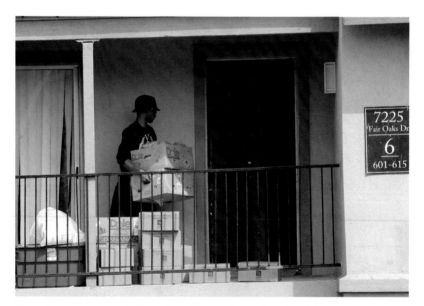

October 2, 2014: Oliver Smallwood carries food from the North Texas Food Bank into the Dallas apartment where he, Louise Troh, Jeffrey Cole, and Timothy Wayne were initially quarantined. (Photo by David Woo, *Dallas Morning News*)

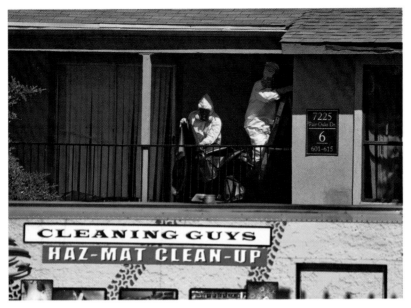

October 3, 2014: workers from CG Environmental-Cleaning Guys decontaminate Louise Troh's Dallas apartment. (Photo by Nathan Hunsinger, *Dallas Morning News*)

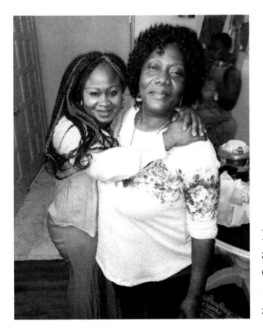

Louise Troh (on right) and her niece Caroline Cargoe. (Courtesy of the author)

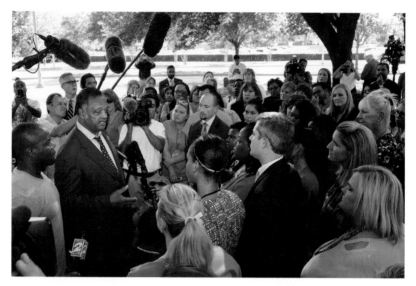

October 7, 2014: Reverend Jesse Jackson visiting Dallas to confer with doctors treating Thomas Eric Duncan, who died the next day. (Photo by Nathan Hunsinger, *Dallas Morning News*)

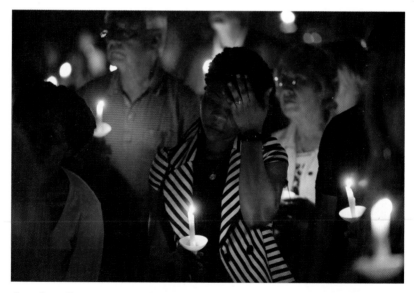

October 8, 2014: Mamie Mangoe, a member of the Dallas Liberian community, at a Wilshire Baptist Church memorial service for Thomas Eric Duncan on the day his death was announced. (Photo by Nathan Hunsinger, *Dallas Morning News*)

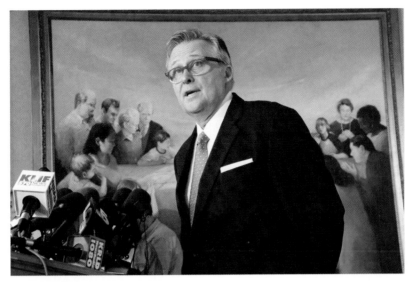

October 8, 2014: Pastor George Mason of Wilshire Baptist Church talks with media about Thomas Eric Duncan. (Photo by Louis DeLuca, *Dallas Morning News*)

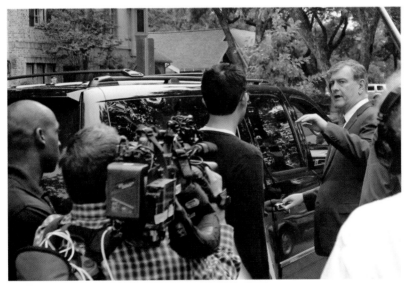

October 12, 2014: Dallas mayor Mike Rawlings is swarmed by media during Dallas's Ebola crisis. (Photo by Louis DeLuca, *Dallas Morning News*)

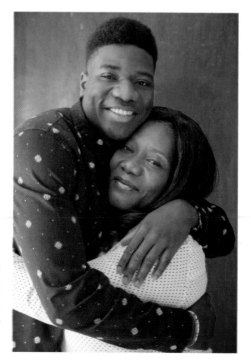

October 23, 2014: Gbor Jallah, Louise Troh's niece (on left), and Youngor Jallah, Louise Troh's daughter, at a protest at Texas Health Presbyterian Hospital Dallas. (Photo by Tom Fox, *Dallas Morning News*)

January 2015: Louise Troh and her son Karsiah Duncan in Dallas. (Photo by Vanessa Gavalya)

Ebola outbreak was in the Dallas news and had been for two months. Kent Brantly, the Fort Worth doctor who was transported from Liberia with Ebola, had recovered almost exactly one month before that and was still in the local news. People from his church were on television, first praying for his recovery and then thanking God for it. He was on the front page of the local newspapers many times. Everyone knew his name and knew that he had been in Liberia treating a terrible outbreak of Ebola.

All I can think is that everyone was afraid when the doctor got Ebola and then relaxed after he recovered.

Or maybe the nurses were just so used to seeing Liberians. Presbyterian is only a few minutes from Vickery Meadow and the hospital gets lots of immigrants. Eric was not the only newly arrived Liberian with a stomachache. Flu season was starting, and people were having lots of allergies with sinus infections that hurt the head. Eric's temperature was bouncing around, not consistently high.

I cannot say why the nurses did not think of Ebola, but I didn't, either. Eric was sick, but he was walking around. Maybe we all thought he didn't look so horrible—not yet.

When Eric gave a sample of his urine, it was darker than normal. It looked purple. I was shocked; I had never seen urine that color. I said, "Why didn't you show me this? When you saw this color, why didn't you let me know?"

After we gave the nurse his urine sample, she took his blood: "In a few days we will give you the results."

But they never did. I did not say anything about the strange urine because they said they would run tests. I thought the tests would tell us what was wrong.

They gave Eric CT scans, looked at his brain and his stomach. They said his brain was all right and his liver was okay. His head pain was still bad. I think the doctor wanted to give him morphine, but I asked them not to. Morphine kills people; I know about it from the nursing home. They give it to people and their breathing is less. Then it gets less and less until they die. Morphine is for hospice. So the nurse gave him extra-strength Tylenol. They also put him on an IV for saline.

We were there for four or five hours. When they took his temperature again, it was 103°. Thirty minutes later, it had dropped to 101.2°. One of the nurses said, "Could be chronic malaria." She said that because she knew he was from Africa.

The doctor asked if Eric was feeling better. The Tylenol had made his headache better, and the saline had hydrated him. Hydration is important in treating fever of all kinds, and it is also the most important thing in treating Ebola. It did make Eric feel better.

Finally, the doctor said Eric had a sinus infection and gave him a prescription for antibiotics he was supposed to take twice on the first day and once a day after that for four days. They told us to go home.

All he needed were antibiotics and Tylenol, they said. Take the medicine, they said to Eric, and you will feel better. We left the hospital at about 4:00 a.m.

What could I have done? I have thought many times about that night. Eric was a gentle man, not one to complain. He was always just thanking everyone for how they were helping him. But I know that complaining is sometimes needed. When the man gave my food away at the UN feeding station in the Ivory Coast, I complained. Even when he swung that stick at my big belly with a baby in it, I kept loudly saying to everyone that my food had been stolen. I would not be quiet. So my food was returned.

When the boss at the food preparation job in Boston would not tell us whether we would be able to work each day until we had already traveled three hours to get to work, I complained. I was new to America. I wanted to work to give my children in Africa the money that would give them food. I didn't want to make the refugee people who had been so good to us mad at me, but I did complain.

If the elderly I care for are not being treated right, I complain. If the schools don't treat one of my sons right, I tell someone. I am a woman with determination. I brought many people from Africa to America. I am an American citizen. I will say if I see wrong.

But I did not complain when they sent Eric home. Many times I go over that night in my mind. I think about the doctor and how he treated us. Was he being careful enough? I saw him look at the information on the computer. He was reading and writing down what we said. I never thought that he wasn't paying attention.

Was he not caring because Eric had no insurance? Was he treating us less than others because we are black? Because we are foreigners? I did not think so. If I saw that, I would have complained. We are the lowly. Nobody cares about us but God. I know that is so. But I don't let fear keep me from saying what is wrong.

Maybe if Eric had been a citizen, that doctor would have wanted more to help him. I am a citizen and have American rights, but Eric did not. But how could I ever know such a thing?

I cannot say the doctor did wrong. Some people are blaming that doctor. I am not. He gave Eric tests. He listened to what Eric said. The only mistake was not seeing that Eric came from Liberia.

But we did not suspect. If we did, I would never have been quiet. If they didn't understand my accent, I would have talked more slowly. I would have talked loudly. I would have stayed in that hospital.

But we did not know that Eric had been around Ebola. He came from a neighborhood where there was no Ebola. There was no Ebola at his work. He was a careful man, not going around people much, not touching them, drinking clean water, going to work and coming home without going in crowds. We had talked every day for weeks. If he had been afraid of Ebola, if he had been seeing Ebola, he would have been talking about it. No one suspected anything.

Eric was planning to go to see his son Karsiah at school on Wednesday. He could not wait until Thanksgiving when Karsiah was coming home. Do you think he would have been demanding to see his son if he could give his son Ebola? Do you think he would have been sleeping with me if he thought he had Ebola? He would not have. If he thought he had the virus, he would have done what my son in Liberia did. He would have gone into a room with water and food and stayed there until he knew.

Some people said later that Eric came to America knowing he had Ebola so that he could get Western medicine treatment. That is a lie and makes no sense. If Eric even thought he might have Ebola, he would have said to Presbyterian doctors that day, "Give me treatment. I am afraid."

Everyone knew that American medicine had cured Kent Brantly. If Eric had such fear, he would have told me, and

I would not have taken him back to my house. I would not have let him wear my son Timothy's jacket. I would not have let my two-year-old grandson Prophet climb onto Eric's lap. I would not have allowed my little granddaughters Rose, Grace, and Knowledge to hug him.

Youngor and I are certified nurse assistants. We work in places with many germs and viruses. Every day after work, we take our shoes off at the door. We do not allow children to touch us before we have washed and changed our clothes. We put our uniforms in a separate basket away from the other clothes. We wash them in the hottest water with disinfectant. We think about the dangers.

Just like Presbyterian nurses and doctors, we did not suspect. Eric and I left the hospital thinking that he had a sinus infection. I was thinking that if Eric was suffering from more than sinus, it would be typhoid fever or malaria, common sicknesses. They were testing his blood. In a few days, we would know the results. They would call us. If Eric needed more treatment, we would know.

Eric and I were tired. I had gone to work at 7:00 a.m. and been up all night. We went home to sleep. We slept together like we always did. When we woke up, we went to get the medicine, and Eric started taking it. He didn't seem to feel as bad as he had. The Ebola virus was growing in him, getting stronger every hour, but we were unaware.

He seemed better. We went on with life, thinking about the future we had waited so long to have. We went to the immigration office to get his papers for work. The official said that Eric could have the papers when the fee of $165 was paid. I didn't have that money.

"I will get that money later when I am paid again," I said. "Then we can get your card, and you will be able to work."

Eric did not need to hear from me about how important working is in America. When he and his brother in Arizona had talked about the life Eric was planning in America, he always talked about how he would work two or three jobs. He was eager to start the life we had been dreaming about for so long. Eric's will to contribute was so strong; he wanted to start making our life good.

I wasn't worried because he had been to the hospital and I trusted the doctors. Eric seemed to feel better. That was our last good day together.

We went by the bank to put my paycheck in. I showed him my paycheck. Liberians think we all make a lot of money. But I don't.

"That's what I get every two weeks," I said.

When Eric saw what the amount was, he just said, "Oh."

"I have to pay my bills out of that," I said. "There isn't much left. When you all are over there, you don't know how we are struggling."

"Everything is going to be all right when I start work," he said. "You are the woman and you are going to keep the paycheck, and we will see what we do with the money. It's going to be all right."

When we walked into the apartment, Eric saw that no one had washed the dishes or run the sweeper. The apartment was not clean.

"Your nephew Oliver is not helping," I said. "He is just eating and then leaving the dishes, not cleaning them." So Eric told Oliver that he should be cleaning up.

"You need to help keep things clean. You know I love to work. I am not feeling well right now, but when I get well I will help you to keep things clean," he said. He was in the apartment for not a week, and he had swept off the porch twice.

"Next time I come home, you will be out washing it with water," I said.

"Yes," he said. "I probably will be."

I sat down in a chair and listened to some music I like on the CD player. I had my head back and my eyes closed, listening. I felt Eric's head resting on my thigh. He'd come over to sit on the floor next to my chair. He started to sing softly about having all the time in the world, but feeling empty because his heart was not full.

As he sang, we both were thinking that those bad days were behind us.

Sometimes when I am awake at night now, sad and suffering, I think about that first visit to the hospital. I wonder if Eric would still be alive if I had not brought him to America. I think that I am to blame. He might still be in Africa, alive. Americans may say that he would have died for sure in Liberia, but not everyone dies of Ebola in Africa. In Liberia, the doctors would have thought of Ebola right away. Eric was a young, strong man, only forty-four years old. They would have given him treatment. It seems so terrible to think that in America he did not get the treatment that would have saved him. But in poor little Liberia, he might have done better.

# CHAPTER NINE

# Calling 911

On Saturday, September 27, when I left for work I was not worried. The hospital checked Eric and soon the antibiotic would work; he would start feeling better.

In the weeks ahead, I would ask myself why I was not suspecting more. I wish I said to everyone, the nurses, the doctor, "Liberia. Liberia. Liberia. He is only six days here from Liberia." I told them twice, once when they were checking us in and later when the nurse came to take more information. I saw them write down what I said. I am usually so alert. I am willing to complain. But I saw nothing for complaints.

Later, experts would say the hospital staff had not trained for how to spot Ebola. The emergency room doctor would say that he hadn't been to any special training. Later, the Centers for Disease Control would show that it sent the hospital a warning about Ebola in August. But the warning said chances were low that Ebola would come to the United States. Doctors should be alert for patients from infected countries, who had come within twenty-one days and who had diarrhea, vomiting, fever, and muscle pain.

"Liberia, Liberia, Liberia. This man is only six days here from Liberia." If I said those words, Eric might be alive today.

But when they answer those questions, who thinks that the doctor will not know what you said? Eric had no diarrhea, no vomiting, and no muscle pain, so I did not suspect. The doctor and the nurses would not have seen such symptoms because he did not have them. The only clear symptom was severe stomach pain, eight on a scale of ten. And that purple urine. They should have tested for Ebola. They didn't.

I went to work early. Before I left, Eric was sitting at the table just looking out the window, looking like he wanted to cry. I wonder now if he was thinking about the pregnant girl he helped. Or maybe not. I don't know what he was thinking, and I knew nothing of the pregnant girl at that time. He was a quiet man. I kissed him good-bye.

He was standing at the top of the stairs when I came home on Saturday. He was more tired than before. Eric was taking the antibiotic each time he was supposed to, but his pain and his weakness were not better. His fever was still present, but when he took Tylenol, it would go down. I kept telling him to drink more water. But he didn't like it.

So when I came home from work I bought him some Gatorade. Gatorade is good to keep you hydrated. He drank a little and left it on the table. Later when I came by and saw it sitting there, I was thirsty. So I drank some of it. Then I put it back on the table. When I saw it again on the table later, it was empty.

"Did you drink this?" I asked Timothy. He told me yes. I never asked Eric if he had poured the Gatorade into a glass or if he had drunk from the bottle. I threw the bottle away. But I wasn't afraid yet. Maybe he hadn't drunk from the bottle. Maybe he wasn't too sick.

On Saturday, he started having some diarrhea. His sister in North Carolina who is a nurse told us that antibiotics sometimes mess with people's stomachs. On that first day, he took two antibiotic pills. So we thought the new problem was because of the antibiotic. What was really happening was that the Ebola virus was growing, and Eric's body was trying to get rid of it. But we didn't know.

We watched TV. I made some food. I was tired, too, so we went to bed early. I was so tired that I just went right to sleep. Once I woke up and he was looking straight into my face. I said, "I'm sorry I'm so sleepy. I have to go to work. I told you about America. It's kind of crazy. I can't be sleepy in my work."

He turned around to the wall then. When I woke again he was looking straight into my face. This time when I opened my eyes, he jumped off the bed and went to the bathroom. I fell asleep again.

When I had a bad dream that woke me up, I saw that he was not in bed. On the floor beside the bed, he had his pants folded under his head so he could use them as a pillow. The belt was on them still, which I thought was strange. Now I realize that he was feeling too sick to be thinking right.

"I am going back and forth to the bathroom so much and the bed is so high. I'm just here."

"Why are you lying on that floor so sorrowful? Here are two pillows," I said, and I got up and put the pillows under his head. Then I found him a sheet. I wish that I had stayed up to help him more, but I could not stay awake. When I woke up to go to work, I put the heavy comforter from the bed over him.

He said, "My stomach is running. I'm not going to mess with that tablet they gave me." So he stopped taking the antibiotics. I had some Tylenol and I wanted him to take it, but his mouth was full of spit. So I brought a plastic bag and had him spit in it. I threw the bag in the trash and sprayed the trash with Lysol and washed my hands, and after wiping my hands I used sanitizer. If he had the flu, I wanted to catch his spit in the plastic instead of on a tissue so the flu virus would not be able to infect anyone.

On my way to work that Sunday morning, I called my daughter Youngor, who works nights and gets off early in the morning. She was on her way home. I asked her if she would stop by my apartment and make Eric some hot Lipton tea. I knew he wouldn't want to drink it because he didn't like hot things, but tea sometimes helps with diarrhea.

When Youngor came into my apartment, Eric was still in the bedroom. He had climbed up into the bed by then, put on his pants, and pulled the comforter over him. She went to the bedroom door to tell him that she would have his tea in the living room, and he should come to get it. She could see that he had on his pants, his socks, and two shirts, but still he was shaking with cold. He told her that he had gone to the bathroom seven times in the night.

"Could you please bring my tea in here? I am so cold," he said. "Can you please give me another blanket?"

She and her cousin Jeffrey jumped into the car and went to Walmart. They bought the heaviest king-size comforter they could find and brought it back for Eric.

When she put the comforter over him, Youngor noticed that Eric's eyes were all red and that he was sweating. She called his sister Mai, the nurse in North Carolina.

Mai asked if Youngor could check his blood pressure and temperature. Youngor went to her car to get the monitors. His blood pressure was high and his temperature was 104°. This number made Youngor very scared.

His sister said, "Is he sitting up? Make him sit up."

So Youngor took his blood pressure and temperature again. They were better but still not good.

"We must go to the hospital," she told Eric.

"Wait until your mother comes home," Eric said. 'I want to drink my tea."

"Okay. You can drink your tea, but then you must go to the hospital. You cannot stay here by yourself," said Youngor. She made him the tea. He let it cool a little like he always did. Youngor could not make him get into the car for the hospital. But she was becoming afraid for his life so she called 911.

"My daddy is going to the bathroom all the time," she told the operator. "He needs to go to the hospital."

When the paramedics came, Youngor stood in the door. "You must have protective clothing. This man is from a viral country," she said. "For safety's sake, don't touch anything."

The men then went back to get gloves and face masks. Youngor didn't say the word Ebola. She only knew that Eric was very sick, and he could have brought something from Africa. Typhoid and malaria are common in Africa, and their symptoms are so much like Ebola that sometimes even doctors have trouble telling what's wrong. Some of the news accounts say that Youngor thought Eric might have Ebola, but she says she did not. Later, other accounts said that even the Centers for Disease Control didn't think there was Ebola at Presbyterian when doctors in Dallas contacted them.

My daughter was being cautious because she is a trained nurse's assistant. She is always cautious and protective of others. She had been reading on the Internet every night for a month about Ebola in Liberia. She thought the paramedics might be afraid of someone who had come from Africa and was sick. Her warning was to make sure they didn't do anything that would make them feel afraid afterward. But for herself and her children who had no protective clothing, she was not yet afraid.

The paramedics could see that Eric did need to go to the hospital. Youngor asked them to put him on a stretcher, but they said they could not carry him down the stairs.

"Can you walk to the ambulance?" one of the paramedics asked.

Eric got up from the bed. He was weak and dizzy, but he could stand on his own. They held his arms so that he would not fall as he walked down the stairs. He was still cold, and they had nothing to cover him. Youngor tried to give them the comforter, but they would not take it.

Youngor did not wait until the ambulance left. Once they had Eric inside, she went toward her own car so that she would be at the hospital when the ambulance arrived. Taking the comforter with her to her red Toyota minivan, she drove to the hospital and went to the desk in the emergency room to give Eric's name. They said he hadn't yet been admitted.

After waiting for a while she asked again. Still no Eric. Youngor called 911 again to ask where Eric was: maybe they took him to another hospital. But no, the operator told her to go to the main desk and to ask if they had admitted him. They didn't have anything, either.

She sat down, putting the comforter on the chair beside her. After about an hour, they told her Eric was in the hospital in Room 42. On the door there she found a sign that said, "Isolation." She was carrying the comforter still, and she asked the nurse if she would give it to Eric. The nurse said no, they would give him blankets.

So Youngor went to my house and folded the comforter over the foot of the bed. Back at her own house, she took off her shoes outside the door, as usual. In addition, she told her children not to touch her. She put her clothes in a bag and sealed it. Then she took a bath with some Clorox in the water. Youngor was listening to her health-worker training and taking extra precautions because they had put Eric in isolation.

I called Eric once from work. No answer. Then I called again—nothing. So I called Youngor, who told me that Eric was in the hospital. When I heard that he was in isolation, I felt my first moment of real fear. In isolation, I would not be able to protect him. What if the doctors were wrong about what they thought he had? They had been wrong about Prophet. But I was able to see Prophet, to touch him and to see for myself how he was doing. If they had Eric in isolation, I would not know this.

I was frightened, but I still thought maybe he had malaria or typhoid fever. When we went to the hospital the first time, when the nurse took Eric's temperature and saw 101°, she had said, "Might be chronic malaria."

I was hoping they put him in isolation because they didn't know what was wrong—just as a precaution. Maybe they would find out what was wrong and then put him in a room where we could visit. I felt protective, of course, because I brought him to America. I knew how alone people can be when they are in America, not like in Africa. I told Eric I would always be with him. Now already he was shut off from me.

When I got off work, Youngor and I went to the hospital. The doctor told me that they were making him comfortable. All they could do was give him liquids and ease his pain. They would test for Ebola, and it would take two days for the results to come back. This was the first time anyone had said "Ebola." I was so frightened, but I kept telling myself that they would think Ebola first because he came from Liberia, where people die from so many other things.

They told us to go to a hallway where there is a big window; we could see Eric there. A nurse was in the room but there was no one else around. I waved at him lying down flat in the bed, shivering. I went to find the nurse to say that he needed a blanket. She told me that he had a fever and did not need one, and that they would take care of Eric. I wasn't allowed to pass him my phone, either. I wanted to tell him that I was sorry, but that I could not get him a blanket.

Then the nurse asked me to leave, even though I told her that I needed to talk to Eric; I didn't think he could hear me through the glass. I wasn't sure she understood my accent. Again she told me that I had to leave.

So we left. I was still hoping to see Eric the next day. I was worried, but I expected the health system to treat him as one of their own. He was approved to come here by the US government; he did not do so illegally. I believed that the doctors would care for him, and that if he had Ebola they would save his life just as they had saved Kent Brantly's.

The hospital called the Dallas County Health and Human Welfare Department that Sunday to say that they might have a patient with Ebola. A woman named Sonya M. Hughes called me the same day to ask me some questions. She wanted to know about Eric's travels and about how he was feeling. I didn't exactly know who she was, but I answered all her questions. I was lucky this woman was working that weekend. She would become a friend to me during the next weeks when I needed friends so much.

Monday before going to work I went to visit Eric again, around 6:15 a.m. I asked at the lobby desk to see Mr. Duncan. She told me to wait. I couldn't go in yet. The nurse who cared for Eric came out.

She said, "It was just the two of us in the ward all night. He is so sweet. I am so sorry he is so sick."

The nurse said, "I gave him some ice to eat and he threw that up."

"Did he vomit?" I asked, and she said, "Only the ice."

"Did he throw up again?" I said.

She said, "No. It was just the ice."

This is not what that nurse told the news media later. I heard her say that Eric had diarrhea so bad that he was sitting on the toilet not able to even leave it. Even with her standing in front of the toilet holding a bag, the vomit was so much that it was going everywhere. One bag would not hold it all and so she had to get other bags, and they all filled up. Maybe she was talking about another night.

The nurse I talked to also said on TV that Eric lied about where he had traveled from, but he did not lie. I think they misunderstood what he told them. When they suspected that Eric might have Ebola, they started to question him, the nurses said later. They asked him if anyone close to him had died recently, anyone in Liberia before he came. He said, "Yes, my daughter died."

I believe he meant my daughter who died in childbirth. He always called my children his children. He was close to her.

Later, when they asked the question again, they asked if he helped the pregnant girl, his daughter who died in childbirth. He said, "Yes, but she was not my daughter." Now he thought they were talking about another person, the landlord's daughter back in Liberia.

The hospital people didn't know about my daughter. So they told people that Eric lied. If anyone had talked to me, I would have told them they were confused. Eric did not lie. But none of them did. They just told wrong stories about a dying man who could not defend himself.

After work on Monday, Youngor and I went back to the hospital. They had moved Eric to a big long room. He was the only person there. I could see him through the glass, and he could hear me. He was lying on his back once again.

"Why don't you sit up? You need to sit up. You will lose your strength if you don't do things for yourself," I said.

"No," he said.

So I said it again louder.

"Sit up." I pushed my palms up to show him that he must pull himself up to sit. But he didn't move.

"No." He was shaking his head. This man had walked to the ambulance. He had gone down the stairs one day ago on his own. Now he was not even able to sit up in bed. What happened? They put him in isolation right away, with no one who loved him to watch what was happening, and now he was so much weaker. Were they giving him food? Were they giving him medicine? The doctor had told me that they were keeping him comfortable. But he was not comfortable.

"You must not do everything these people tell you just because they say so," I said. "You must keep your strength. Don't be afraid to tell them what you want to do." He was so easygoing. He would not fight to get his own way. All day I was thinking that I would not be able to protect him the way I had protected my grandson Prophet when they wanted to take his liver.

Eric was alone, with no one who loved him to watch out. I know from the nursing home that people who stay in bed lose all their strength fast. We were separated by walls and windows, doors that wouldn't open. I wanted to stay with Eric to watch over him and make sure he wasn't cold. He had no human to touch him. No one to ask questions. He would have to protect himself. But I couldn't get him to sit up and keep his strength.

"You don't have to do what they say," I told him through the glass. "You must be thinking for yourself." I was talking loud.

A nurse heard me then. "You must leave here," she said. I knew she didn't like what I was saying to Eric.

But I had to protect him. I didn't care that she didn't like me. He would soon be alone; I needed him to be strong.

"Go on, now," the nurse said. "We have security if you don't leave."

I saw that she had called a security guard who was coming toward us.

"Come on, let's leave for now," Youngor said.

So I waved good-bye at Eric. He moved his hand to wave a little at me. I thought I would come back again the next day when another nurse was around. I am around nurses all the time. Some are good. Some are bad.

I never thought that those few minutes looking at him through the glass would be the last time I saw his face. I would have looked much longer to remember just how he looked. I would have stood there until the guard pushed me away. But I didn't know.

I never saw Eric again.

He called his mother in North Carolina that day. She told me that he was crying, bitterly. He said, "I can't see anybody. I'm just here alone in a dark room. They are hurting me. They are hurting me all over my body. They only come running into here and draw my blood. They spill my blood. It is all over the floor."

She told me, "He is crying just like a baby."

# CHAPTER TEN

# Diagnosis: Ebola

Tuesday, September 30, I was at the Laundromat washing clothes when a doctor from the hospital called. She said the Ebola test results would be ready in forty-five minutes and she would call me. I was folding clothes, waiting. The phone rang a couple of times. The doctor told me thirty minutes. I kept folding clothes.

Then she called and said it would be fifteen minutes. I kept folding, smoothing out the warm towels, pressing T-shirts with my hands until all the wrinkles were flattened, shaking out pillowcases. These were Timothy's clothes and mine. I did not have Eric's clothes with me. This is calm work. It helped to keep my body doing quiet things. No word is scarier than "Ebola."

I was thinking, *Of course they will say he has Ebola. On the second visit to the hospital the nurse said, "You come from an infected country." So they will say Ebola even if it isn't.*

The phone rang again. It was the doctor. She sounded very grim. "I am sorry to say that the test shows Mr. Duncan to have the Ebola virus."

When I heard the word "Ebola," my mind wanted to say that the doctor was wrong. All the reasons I hadn't suspected went through my mind. They took his temperature at the airport many times. He walked from the apartment to the ambulance. No vomiting. No bleeding. My mind was defending against this news. And then I remembered that purple color in his urine when I first took him to Presbyterian. Why didn't the doctors see that? The doctors make mistakes. Maybe this Ebola diagnosis was a mistake. I couldn't believe this terrible news.

My body was cold with fear. I remembered how cold Eric was before he went to the hospital. I wondered if the cold was the beginning of his sickness. Would he die?

Would I die, too? Would my family all die?

I was so afraid that my mind wouldn't work. I didn't know what to do. I wanted to go home where people couldn't see me. I gathered my clothes together, put them in the car, and drove toward home. I couldn't think about what might come next.

I needed to go to the grocery for food because we didn't have enough at the apartment. But I didn't stop. I didn't want to be outside my apartment. What would people do if they knew that my fiancé was the one with Ebola? They would run away from me. They would look at me with fear. They would hold their children tightly. At the Ivy Apartments where I lived there was no one in the parking lot in the middle of the day. I hurried to get my clean clothes inside.

Soon, photos of the Ivy Apartments would be everywhere. Pictures of my closed door would be shown to all the world. I didn't know that then; I had no idea what was about to happen.

Inside, signs of Eric were all over the place: the mattresses where he had slept; chairs he sat in. I looked at the table and remembered the bottle of Gatorade there. Eric drank some and I'd had some, too. Later, Timothy came by and drank the rest. I hadn't wanted to think about that, but now I was thinking about these things all the time.

In the bedroom were Eric's clothes and the bed where we had made love and talked about the happy life we were about to have. In the bathroom were the towels and washcloths he had used. The toilet where he had diarrhea was one we all used. I cleaned it with Clorox on Sunday after his night of diarrhea; now I would clean it again.

I looked at the knobs on the sink where he turned on water to wash his hands. I looked at the knobs on the sink in the kitchen where he got water to drink: the doorknobs, the light switches, and the mattresses my grandchildren slept on; Timothy's jacket that Eric wore to keep warm. I was happy to think of how particular Timothy was. He did not wear that jacket again when he saw Eric wear it. Karsiah's clothes that I had loaned Eric were now dangerous, too. The virus could be anywhere.

But I calmed myself. I know about viruses. I work around them every day. Keeping things clean is the important part. On the Internet I read that the Ebola virus can only live six hours in the air on a dry surface, though it might live longer on something wet. The CDC website says that in a body fluid, the virus can stay for days at room temperature. Youngor and I did not get training on Ebola where we worked in nursing homes, so we did our own research.

So maybe the spit I cleaned from Eric's mouth could have Ebola in it. I threw the bag in the trash. I washed my hands with disinfectant. I know how to wash hands so that no virus can be left. Ebola can only spread through contact with skin or other human membranes.

I put on gloves and picked up the clothes Eric wore. There were T-shirts, some pants, and some underwear. I gathered the towels and washcloths he had used. One was my favorite brown towel that one of my daughters bought me. It's just the right size and feels right to use when I rinse myself off. He liked it also. It's my favorite. I left it out of the bag, and later washed it out with disinfectant and hot water. Then I let it dry. From the CDC site I knew that any virus remaining would die on the dry surface.

I sprayed everything else with Mean Green and then with Clorox and put it all in a bag that I sealed tightly. Then I put two more bags over that and sealed them. His suitcases were still sitting in the bedroom. He hadn't been wearing his own clothes since that first day. He had been wearing Karsiah's clothes and sometimes Timothy's jacket. So those clothes of his hadn't been taken out of the suitcase. He didn't have a temperature when he packed them. Even if he had Ebola, he wasn't contagious until he began to show symptoms.

So I zipped the suitcase and closed the satchel. I put them in the corner and sprayed all over and around with disinfectant. Then I sprayed the bed with Clorox. Later, people would say so much about those sheets and pillows still being on the bed for days afterward. Yes, I left them there, but they dried out for a day, then I sprayed them with Clorox, and they dried again. Maybe Eric wasn't even contagious.

The amount of virus in the blood determines whether Ebola is contagious. In Africa, a most dangerous time for catching Ebola is after the person has died. Before symptoms show up, the virus is too low to infect. After it kills a person, the body is full of virus. People who wash the body, prepare it for burial or burning can get Ebola easily then.

Eric did not throw up while he was at my house. He did not have diarrhea until he took those antibiotics. I still thought it could be that he had malaria or maybe typhoid fever. I knew that doctors can be wrong. I kept remembering that two years ago, the doctors had said my grandson Prophet was going to die in two weeks, but he was still alive and doing great. Doctors can be wrong. But even if they weren't, Eric might not have passed the virus to us. My mind was moving so fast now, going one place and then the other. I was afraid, and then telling myself not to be afraid. My breathing would be fast and then my heart would beat so fast, too.

The phone rang: it was the school telling me that a policeman would bring my son Timothy home. In a few minutes, the phone rang again. It was the school saying that I would have to come and get my son. Sonya from the Health Department had called the school on Monday just to check with the nurse on how Timothy was feeling. She did not mention Eric or Ebola. But by Monday reporters had told the world that a patient at Presbyterian who had recently come from Liberia was being tested for Ebola. By Tuesday afternoon, when the diagnosis came in, all the media did stories saying Ebola was in Dallas. Then Eric's name was released.

The media quickly found out that Thomas Eric Duncan had come to visit Louise Troh. Soon they would find his picture on Facebook: Eric looking solemn in a bright green shirt would soon be one of the most famous photos in the world. But they never showed any pictures of Eric in the hospital. Later, when the nurses who cared for Eric got sick, they showed pictures of them and gave messages from them; but for Eric, there was nothing.

I am grateful they did not find a photo of me. If my face had been on the television or the papers, I would have felt like a criminal. Already I felt that people thought I had done something wrong. But I am innocent. We were both innocent.

Even without my picture or my name, it was not hard for the school nurse to figure out what was happening. So I went to the school, where I found Timothy at the school nurse's office. He didn't understand what was happening. He asked me why he was going home with me instead of walking as usual. When we got to the car, I told him that Eric had Ebola.

Timothy said, "I don't have Ebola."

Then he was quiet for a minute. He said, "Wow. Do you think we're going to get Ebola?"

I said, "Well, let's give it to God."

When I got home the phone rang again. It was the Dallas County Health Department.

"Where is Eric's stuff? We need to know," the person said.

"It's in the room."

"Stay away from the room."

"Why should I stay away from the room? I've been using this room, lying in this bed, I've been using the bathroom. It makes no sense. I have been sleeping in this room since he came."

"Just don't sleep there," the person said. "Do you have a temperature? Do you feel hot or cold?"

"No. I am fine."

"Who is living with you in the house?"

"My two nephews and my son."

"Are they home now?"

By this time Oliver and Jeffrey had come in. So I said yes.

"How are they feeling?"

I didn't know, but they looked fine. So I said, "They are good."

"Don't let them leave the house. Do you understand? No one is to leave. We will come over to take your temperature. Stay away from each other. Do not touch each other. Do you understand?"

"Yes, I understand."

Then she asked me to tell her everyone who had been around Eric. There were not that many, maybe not even ten, because we had mostly stayed home.

I told the health worker that I had been about to go grocery shopping and that we had almost no food in the house. She said they would bring us food. When she asked what we wanted, the boys said burritos. But the Health Department didn't bring anything. We waited all day and no food.

They said that Timothy, my nephews, and I were supposed to stay in our house for twenty-one days. They said, "Don't go out at all," and they would come to take our temperature. If our temperatures went up over 100°, it could mean that we had Ebola. We would be contagious only when our temperatures went up. There was no set mark that would mean Ebola for sure. But a temperature was the best way to know if the virus was growing enough to make us sick and infect other people. If we had no symptoms, we were not contagious.

Eric had a temperature when we took him to the hospital the first time, and they sent him home. I had slept with him when he had a temperature. We made love three nights with no protection. He had held my grandchildren. When did he become contagious? If temperature was the true test, he could have been passing the virus to us all as early as Wednesday, the day when I first noticed that his skin was hot. He was sick enough to go to the hospital on Thursday. He told the doctor his pain was an eight on a scale of ten. Ebola was causing that pain.

Was he contagious as we sat in the waiting room, while he lay with his head on my lap? Was he shedding the virus through his saliva and sweat when we returned home and slept together for three more nights? On Saturday night, did he wash his hands every one of those seven times he went to the bathroom with diarrhea? Eric was a careful man, but he did not have my training.

I was too sleepy to listen for the water running. I remembered those times when I awakened on Saturday night to find him staring into my face, breathing into my face, his eyes looking so sad. When I held the plastic bag to his mouth Sunday morning to take away the spit, was Ebola virus wiggling all through it? And the Gatorade that we shared: I couldn't let my mind think of the Gatorade my son and I drank after Eric had tasted it.

Eric was with us, very sick, until Sunday—five days. I thought of Youngor, my calm, beautiful, responsible, first-born daughter, who had told the emergency medical technicians to put on gloves and masks, who had no gloves or mask, holding the thermometer to his mouth, pulling it from his lips with spit coating the glass, holding it to the light, leaning near to check it. Taking his temperature once and taking it again. Holding his arm to check his blood pressure. Was his skin wet with sweat? Even the tiniest cut on her hand would let the virus in. If she wiped her eyes, touched her nose, scratched an itch, she might die.

We all might die. If I kept thinking of such things, I would be afraid and then all my family would be afraid. As Youngor had told the doctors when I decided that her baby Prophet would not have a liver transplant, "In African culture, our parents can decide for us. So whatever her decision is, we are going to go by that." What I decided would guide my family.

I had made many decisions in the face of fear. I had brought my family out of war and exile. I rescued them from violence and hunger. I had run from the soldiers with my just-delivered baby and with my hands holding my stomach still big from childbirth. Later, when the blood-covered man beaten by the soldiers called to me for help, I answered, yes, I knew him; and I refused to kill that man when the soldiers told me to.

My family would be watching me now. I decided then that I must not believe we were going to die. I decided that Eric would get better. None of us would get sick. And we would all have the wonderful life we planned for.

In that decision, I had the help of God—and the help of Timothy. In the coming weeks, it would be Timothy who refused to give in to fear. He would dry my tears and put his arms around me. While a whole city, a whole country panicked, Timothy, just thirteen, would handle his fear like an African warrior from the greatest legends of our people, with no reproach, only courage.

Timothy began his fight against fear that Wednesday as we drove home from school. When I told him that we had to stay inside for twenty-one days, he said, "I don't have Ebola. I'm going to school tomorrow. How do you know Uncle Eric has Ebola?"

"They say he does," I said.

"I'm going to school tomorrow," he said. "They aren't talking about me. The school nurse told me I can come back. So I can go. You didn't understand what they were saying to you."

"No, Timothy," I said. "I'm sorry, but you can't."

When we got home, Youngor called me to say that I needed to get rid of all the bedding.

"I don't want to throw away that new blanket that you bought," I told her.

"That blanket is not as important as your life," Youngor said. She was frightened for me. "I don't know what's gone on at that house, but we need to be careful and preserve your life."

Youngor went to Walmart to buy a foam mattress and a comforter for me to sleep on. Then we cleaned everything. We had two big jugs of Clorox that we used to wash everything. We took the bedding and the sheets and washed them in Clorox. We sprayed everywhere germs could live.

We kept working until Timothy said, "Please, I can't stand this smell of chlorine. My eyes are hurting. Can you stop?" So we did.

Next to the four of us, Youngor and her children had been most exposed to Eric. The Health Department visited her apartment. Cameras were outside her apartment at 4:00 a.m. that Wednesday morning. Reporters were knocking on the door. When the Health Department saw how many reporters were around, the health worker said they could move her and her family, but Youngor didn't want to be moved.

"Is it safe here?" the health worker asked.

"No, but we're staying," Youngor said. They said that she and her family would stay inside for a week or so and if they did not have any symptoms, they could go out. They would still need to take their temperatures every day, but they could go to work.

Youngor could work, but she could not work with patients. Her work would have to be in the office. Youngor is careful. She did not want to infect anyone. Her fiancé, Aaron, had not been around Eric much so he went back to work. But Youngor and her children stayed inside for the full twenty-one days.

The next morning was Wednesday. That morning I didn't have to call Timothy to get out of bed. He got up and took his shower early. I told him that he must stay inside, but he said again that I didn't understand what people were saying. He walked out the door and off to school.

In a little while the school called. They said, "You have to come and get Timothy. He can't stay here."

So I went again to the school. At the office, they were whispering. I heard someone say, "Her husband has Ebola." Then they laughed. Laughing? This was the first of many times when I would wonder why people were acting so mean. There was another boy in the office, trying to hear everything, and they told him to go away.

Timothy was mad and would not talk to me. I remembered how he hadn't wanted to welcome Eric. I had brought this danger on him. It was a terrible thing. I should have told Eric not to come until Ebola was gone from Liberia. But his neighborhood was not infected. His temperature was not high when he left Liberia. Again and again I repeated these things to myself. Now it was too late to protect my youngest son or anyone else in my family who had been around Eric.

"I am sorry. There is nothing I can do about it, Timothy," I said. These were my first apologies to Timothy. There would be many more.

We went straight home. At the Ivy Apartments, reporters were all around in the parking lot setting up their cameras. They didn't know who I was, but maybe they knew where I lived because Eric put my address on the hospital forms. They didn't notice me until I went to my door; then they were all looking and pointing. I didn't want to talk with them. I went into my apartment, shut the door, and locked it. I pulled the curtains so that no one could see in. And then I turned and saw the picture I put on the wall with thumbtacks. It was Jesus praying on his knees in the Garden of Gethsemane. Light was shining down on him.

Timothy went right to his room. He was so angry, and he did not want to believe it. By then five of the schoolchildren in our family had been told that they should not come back to their schools. Some parents at my grandchildren's schools were not bringing their children to school, and others were coming to take them home early. Students were frightened and afraid to touch one another.

On Wednesday, Stanley Gaye called. He is the president of the Liberian Community Association of Dallas/Fort Worth.

"You don't know me," he said. "But I'm calling you to see if there's any help that we can give you. Your Liberian brothers and sisters are standing by to help you."

I was glad to hear from Stanley because I was feeling very alone. I had been having people calling for hours, people who I thought were friends of mine, people I had helped in many ways. Some of them were thinking that I had Ebola, and that I would soon be dead. I knew they thought this because they were talking to me in very rude ways. They didn't think I would be around too long and so they could say anything. They were not thinking about Eric or my family, just themselves.

"Isn't our life hard enough already?" some Liberians would say to me as if I had done something wrong to them. "Why did you bring that man here?" and "Why did that man come to infect America? He should have stayed in Liberia. Now everyone will hate us."

By now many reporters had my number and were trying to get me to say things. I had never talked with a reporter in my life. I was so afraid to say something wrong. I was suspicious of everyone. So when Stanley Gaye called, I thought, "What does he want?"

"How are you doing?" Stanley said. "What can we do for you?"

I had no requests so I didn't stay on the phone long that day. I could have asked for some food but I didn't think of that. But Stanley would keep calling, trying to help me through the quarantine. Already many people were talking about how I needed a lawyer. I didn't know anything about that. Some people were saying that I was not Eric's wife, and so I would have no standing in a lawsuit, but some lawyers said that under Liberian community law, I was Eric's wife and could sue.

A friend of my daughter Nopie called to say she knew a woman from Washington, DC, a Liberian named Saymendy Lloyd who runs a group that helps women and could help me get a lawyer.

"I want to be the one who speaks out for you," Saymendy said when she called me. "I can call Jesse Jackson to see if he will help you."

I said okay. Maybe I needed him to stand up for me.

When I looked out the window, I saw a sheriff's car parked facing our door. When Sonya Hughes from the Health Department and a person from the Centers for Disease Control tried to come to see us, they couldn't get to our apartment because of all the reporters and the security guards who had been hired to protect the property. The health workers were dressed like anyone else.

When they walked into the parking lot, which the sheriffs were guarding, the reporters asked, "Who are you? If you're reporters, we're going in with you. You can't go if we can't go."

But the health workers wouldn't talk to them. They didn't want the reporters knowing who they were because they knew the reporters would never leave them alone, and they couldn't answer questions. One reporter climbed the fence and ran after the health workers. He came up the stairs and when the health workers knocked on the door, he was right outside with them.

When I answered the door, Sonya told me to shut it. She didn't want the reporter to see inside. The security guards saw what was happening and came to take the reporter away.

Then I let the health workers in. They asked us questions. They took our temperatures. They gave us each our
own thermometer, the kind you put under your arm. The
Health Department had trouble deciding which thermometer to use. First was that one that you put under your arm.
Later they gave us the old-fashioned kind that you stick under your tongue and wait for a few minutes. The health
officials gave us lessons in how to place the thermometer
under our tongues and how long to leave it in. Then they
came back with newer thermometers that go under the
tongue but register temperature faster. When the monitor
is as high as it's going to go, the thermometer dings.

They asked me to make sure I had told them everyone
who was in contact with Eric. They said they'd heard that we
had a big party and that maybe a hundred people came to it.

I said, "No, we didn't have a party. Who told you that?"

They said people in the Liberian community said so. But
it wasn't true. There had been no party. I had spent so much
money on my Liberian daughter's funeral. I had borrowed
money for Eric to come. I didn't even have money for us to
marry. How would I have money for a party? My family and
just a few friends had met Eric. Eric's son Karsiah, who was
270 miles away at Angelo State University, had never been
able to see his father. He had talked to his father on the
phone but nothing more.

The health workers asked if I had traveled to Liberia to
be with Eric before he left the country. I had not been anywhere near Africa in sixteen years. I use any money I have
for plane tickets to help people come from Africa to America. Nobody from America goes back to Africa if they don't
have a house to live in. I did not go back to Liberia because

I had no money for that. Why did people make up these crazy stories?

The Health Department people said they heard that we had people from the church come into our apartment to pray for Eric. We had not. No one from the church came to our house, and we did not go to church on the first Sunday he was here. I had to work both Sundays. Lies, lies, lies: these Liberians are telling so many lies that I told the Health Department people I didn't want to hear any more.

"Don't listen to anyone else. When anyone tells you anything, just take down their number and give it to me," I said. "Then I will call them and make it straight."

That evening, a sheriff's deputy named Michael Monnig came to the apartment with some papers that said we were not allowed to leave for twenty-one days. They said we would be charged with a crime if we did. All four of us promised to stay inside.

A week later, the sheriff's deputy started having stomach pain and felt tired. He went to a Care Now clinic. People at the clinic called 911 saying they had a man who had contact with Patient Zero. Patient Zero is what they started calling Eric. The clinic was closed and sealed off. Everyone was sent home. The sheriff's black SUV was sealed with tape by hazmat teams. This deputy never even saw Eric. The deputy barely came in the apartment. He did not touch anyone or anything. People were going so crazy.

A paper telling about Ebola was put on all the doors at the Ivy Apartments. Our apartment did not get one. No one would come near our door.

At the end of that day, Wednesday, the Health Department brought us some bottled water and sandwiches. They

were ham sandwiches wrapped in plastic. Ugly food—and
that was all they brought.

I called Max from the Open Bible Sunday-school class
to tell him what happened. I asked if the class would pray
for my family, and he said that they would. He must have
called Pastor George because the pastor called me a little
while later to say that God would be with me, and not to be
afraid. He said that my church would stand with me and
help me. And then we prayed on the phone. Later he sent a
letter to the church telling everyone at the church that they
were safe. No one from my family had been to church since
Eric arrived in the country. Pastor George asked everyone
to pray for us.

By the third day, Thursday, October 2, even more reporters camped outside. We were all feeling so crowded. Not
even the windows were open. We couldn't take the trash
out. We couldn't go outside to go to the dumpster, and if
we did, everyone would think our trash was infected. So
we lived with it. Once Oliver opened the door to make a
phone call but he didn't go past the doorway. He stood just
on the inside of the chalk drawings of a house and a heart
that my granddaughters had made on the concrete outside
our door. He finished his call and waved to the news media.

We could hear helicopters. More police officers were
standing in the parking lot now to keep the reporters away.
Reporters were bribing our neighbors to let them use their
apartments. One reporter got into an apartment near us
and refused to leave even when the resident said go away.
He had to call the manager. Some of the reporters acted
like they were pizza delivery people so they could get
nearer to our apartment. At the end of the day, the mayor

of Dallas, Mike Rawlings, talked to the news media and told them they had to behave better.

The Health Department was tracking down people who might be infected. I was getting phone calls from my loved ones, who were being told they must be in quarantine. Even the ones who had little contact with Eric were told they must avoid contact with others and take their temperatures two or three times a day.

On the television there was just bad news and more bad news. Binyah Kesselly, chairman of the Liberia Airport Authority Board of Directors, said that if Eric returned to Liberia he would be prosecuted for lying on a health form before he departed. But he did not lie. When the reporters called, I told them Eric didn't do anything wrong. I told them the truth, but nobody was listening.

Since Monday, I'd tried to talk to Eric on the phone, but every time I called they said that doctors were in with him, or tests were being done, and to call back. Then when I called back, the phone would ring and ring, but no one would pick up. On Thursday morning, he answered.

"How are the children?" he asked.

"Are you walking around?" I asked.

"How can I be walking around? I have all these machines on me," he said. He said he had had a good night. His fever had gone down.

Then he said, "Oh, let me get off this phone. They are coming. I have to go."

He said he would call me back, but he did not.

Then I saw the report on television about how Eric helped the pregnant girl in his neighborhood. People had started dying of Ebola after Eric left. The reporters were discussing whether Eric knew the girl had Ebola. So I called Eric again, and again he picked up the phone.

"I saw on the screen about that pregnant girl you helped in Monrovia," I said.

"You don't know anything about that," he said. "If anyone asks you about that, you tell them to talk to myself."

"I am not mad at you about that girl," I said. "I am just wanting you to get well."

This was true; I was thinking all the time about Eric getting well. But I was also mad that he had not told me about that girl. He was a good man to help her, and I know from all news accounts that no one had Ebola in that neighborhood, and that no one got sick with Ebola until after Eric left. He had his visa weeks before he helped the pregnant girl.

Eric should not have kept it secret from me that he helped the pregnant girl. He was not sick when he arrived. But maybe if he had told me about the girl, we would have figured out that he was getting ill from helping her. I was angry now, so angry that he exposed many people to danger, even though he didn't know why he was getting sick. He took my grandchildren in his lap. I cannot forgive that he did not tell me the truth about the girl. It might have made a difference. Right then I thought that once he got well, I would sit him down at the table and tell him how wrong he had been. And I would tell him to go away.

# CHAPTER ELEVEN

# Men in Yellow Suits

In those days my Liberian friends wanted to organize a vigil outside Presbyterian Hospital with candles and some singing so that maybe Eric would hear of it and know that people were caring for him. But they could not get any others to come near the hospital. People were saying that the hospital did not know what to do about Ebola. Maybe they didn't know how to keep it from spreading. Maybe someone would just go there to visit someone and touch something and come away with Ebola. Not only Liberians thought this. Other people did, too, and stopped going to Presbyterian.

Presbyterian Hospital even closed its emergency room for some days. The ambulance that took Eric to the hospital was not being used anymore. It had to be cleaned. The workers who picked Eric up were in voluntary quarantine. A homeless man who was carried in the ambulance was also put in quarantine.

Always before, Liberians in the United States were worried about their relatives in Africa getting Ebola. Everyone had terrible stories to tell, sometimes about whole families dying. Now these Dallas Liberians were getting calls from their Liberian relatives who were worried about them.

My neighborhood, Vickery Meadow, usually has many volunteers coming to help the immigrants who live there. But now the volunteers were afraid and staying away, the news said. At Heart House, where children come to get help with reading and math, volunteers were not coming. At Healing Hands, the medical clinic, nurses were not coming to work. Even people who needed food were afraid to come to the food bank.

Three men who lived in Ivy Apartments, where I lived, were told to leave work when the boss saw where they lived. In the Dallas newspaper, a man named Jason Nancarrow wrote a letter that expressed sympathy for our situation but said that "the system is broken."

He added: "The root of this crisis is Vickery Meadow. You can't stuff that many poor immigrants, refugees and undocumented aliens together and then look away, as this city has been doing. Vickery Meadow is a boiling pot that will spill over again if we keep ignoring it."

Eric never was around any of the places in Vickery Meadow where people were so afraid. No one who met Eric was around those places. People were just acting crazy. Eric had been in the hospital since Sunday. According to the CDC, the Ebola virus dies in several hours if it is not in a moist place. How could they get it?

So when someone from Anderson Cooper's show on CNN called me and asked me to talk with him, I said yes. I wanted to stop all these lies. I said to Anderson that I told people at Presbyterian Hospital on our first visit that Eric was from Liberia. I told him that Eric did not tell me anything about being exposed to Ebola. I told him that yes, the sheets that Eric slept on were still on the bed, but we were sleeping in the living room. I was taking everyone's temperatures every hour.

For two days, we got by on what food I still had in the house. Finally, the Red Cross and the food bank brought some more food for us to cook. They left the boxes of food outside the door. No delivery person wanted to come inside. They wouldn't be allowed. And they would be afraid of us.

But when my nephews drank the orange juice, they got a stomachache. I looked on the package and saw that the juice was outdated. They brought us old food. They also brought canned food. Africans like fresh food. I don't eat canned food if I can find any other food. Finally, a Jewish charity brought us some dishes of good food.

Since Tuesday, no one except the Health Department people had come to see us. They told us that we couldn't even touch each other or sit by each other. Nobody who came in was supposed to get closer than three feet from us. Oliver and Jeffrey, who I always call my "nephews," were so afraid of me that they were wearing gloves.

If my phone rang, they would pick it up with a paper towel to hand to me. Then they would throw the towel away. They didn't want me to touch any dishes they ate from, so they had their own bowls and spoons that they washed and then took to their room.

Oliver said he didn't want me touching his food at all. So I said, "Okay, cook your own food."

But Oliver doesn't know how to cook. He can't make rice or soup. He made a mess, and nobody could eat what he cooked. So he said, "Okay. You can cook my food but I will get it out of the pots."

"So when I put food in the pot, Ebola goes away?" I said. "But when I dip it out, Ebola comes back?" I laughed.

But Timothy would not obey the rules. He would come up to me and put his hands all over me and say, "I am not touching. I am not touching." He would eat the food I fixed and sit as close to me as he could.

"You do not have Ebola," he would say. "I do not have Ebola, either." Sometimes he would try to eat from the same fork I was using. I told him no, but then he would put his fork on my plate and eat my food.

Then he would say again, "You do not have Ebola."

That boy loves me so much. I could not keep him away from me. I didn't have a temperature, so I knew he would not catch Ebola from me. I did not think I had it at all. But if I did, I would have to just trust in God. The only way to keep Timothy from me would have been to tie him up.

Friends and relatives were calling me all the time to tell me what the news media were saying. The whole country was getting frightened and angry. People on television were saying that no one from viral countries should be allowed to come to the United States. People who live outside Dallas were telling my friends that they did not want to come to Dallas. Dentists were asking patients if they had been near anyone who had Ebola. Dallas schools where my son and my grandchildren went to classes were being scrubbed out. Some parents wouldn't let their children come to school. I read in the newspaper that people were asking African children if they were Liberian. When they said yes, these people where telling the Liberian children to stay away from them.

People on the Internet were saying that we were terrorists, and Eric brought Ebola to America so everyone would be afraid and die. Such foolish things. Hearing those things hurt me. And they made me afraid. I knew that people could do terrible things to my family if they started thinking of us in bad ways.

Later, one of the nurses who took care of Eric said that one day Eric was well enough to watch television, and he saw what bad things people were saying about him. His face looked so shocked that she said she told him maybe it would be good to watch something else.

On Thursday night at about 11:00 p.m., I was on the comforter where I slept in the living room. Timothy was curled up with a cushion. I was facing the wall thinking my life was so terrible. I was so worried about Eric and so hoping no one else would get Ebola. Someone knocked at the door—a nice polite knock. People were not being so polite all the time.

One of the health workers who came to see us banged on the door rudely, like a policeman or some criminal about to bust in. This was not any way to treat us. He didn't have a right to do that. So I told him that he must act better and not be so demanding with his pounding on the door like he was going to break it down.

Then the health worker stopped being rude and said, "Yes, ma'am." Next time, he knocked more nicely.

Even though this 11:00 p.m. knock was a respectful knock, after 11:00 is not a respectful time. So I didn't get up. Jeffrey answered the door. Light came flooding through the apartment when Jeffrey opened the door. The reporters had seen that the health workers and the county judge were outside knocking and had turned their floodlights toward our apartment. They were hoping to get a photo of one of us, but Jeffrey stayed behind the door.

A man poked his head around the door. I looked around. This was a face everyone in Dallas had seen on television: serious, pale-skinned, red-brown hair. This man looked as different from Liberians as anyone could.

"Hello, Louise. I'm County Judge Clay Jenkins," he said. "I'm sorry to be coming so late. How are you?"

I was feeling low. I was wishing so much that I could have my old life back. But when the judge spoke to me so politely, I came to my senses and got up. I sat in a chair and he stood looking around. The room was dark. The television was off because it was broken. No sofas, just chairs, tables, and mattresses. Timothy and I sleeping on the floor. It was a sad place.

I knew this man as a good friend to people who needed help. Last summer, when 50,000 children from Central America came over the Texas-Mexico border, lots of people were so mad. They wanted the children sent right back. But this man said Dallas County would make room for thousands of them. He started looking for places they could stay until the courts could do something with them. When he found a warehouse and some vacant schools, he went to talk to the neighbors who lived near. When he told them what he wanted, they agreed to have the children close by. But other people were even madder at the refugee children and the judge. Some picketed his house.

These people who picketed his house were so strange. They held signs that said things like, "American Rights for Americans Only." Some were people who think Texas should be its own nation, not part of America. I didn't even want these kinds of people to know my name. I knew that coming to help us would cause the judge more trouble with such people. And it did. A few days after he visited me, people would picket his daughter's elementary school, protesting that she was in class after her daddy had visited us.

But that night, all the judge was thinking about was that I was sleeping on the floor. "I'm unhappy that you are still here," the judge said.

What did he mean? I couldn't go anywhere. Even if I was allowed, I hadn't thought about moving. Where would I go? Who would move my stuff? Everyone was afraid of me and all my things. I didn't have money to rent a place. I couldn't get past the sheriff's car sitting outside my apartment. They would put me in jail if I even tried to leave. They told me they would.

I didn't know it then, but the judge was also worried about us still being in the apartment with the sheets on my bed, and the bags of clothes and towels that I had sprayed with Clorox. He was thinking about how the body begins trying so hard to shed the Ebola virus as it begins to invade the blood in bigger and bigger numbers. He was thinking that a man with a fever would be sweating as he tossed and turned in the bed. His sweat and flakes of his skin might be filled with virus. The CDC had first said the things that Eric had been in contact with were toxic but at a low risk level. Then they changed and said things that Eric had used were the highest level of toxic substances, the most dangerous.

For two days the judge had been trying to find a company that would come to our apartment and clean out the contaminated things. But nobody wanted the job. These companies clean up AIDS patients' rooms and all sorts of other places where there is danger of sickness being spread. But they said that their clients might hear that they had been around Ebola and be afraid to use them anymore. They also said that once they had all the material out of our apartment, there was nowhere to go with it. No landfill would agree to take it.

Finally, the judge found a company to do the job. The cleaners' trucks had pulled up to streets around our apartment and were waiting in their yellow hazmat suits that night. They were ready to begin disinfecting and throwing things away.

But the judge heard they were waiting and said, "We can't clean the apartment with Louise and her family still in it." So he sent the trucks away.

Then the judge came to see us. "We need to get you another place to stay. I'm going to look for a place. Then I will take you there myself," said the judge. "I'm going to take care of you like you were my own family. Don't worry about anything."

This kindness made me want to cry. I was lying on the floor, feeling like nobody was thinking well of me or wanting to help me. And then the judge came. He is a godly man. Maybe he was so kind because he had misfortune, too. When he was a seven-year-old boy his father had a heart attack when he was with his son in a Dallas park and later died.

Then on Thanksgiving Day twenty-two years ago, the judge had a terrible car wreck. His car skidded on a patch of ice and jumped a median into traffic coming toward him. He broke his neck and other bones. His brain was injured, and he was bleeding a lot inside. It took him three years to get well enough to work at his job as a lawyer again. The judge started going to church and praying to God. He started helping homeless people and others in need. Then he ran for county judge so he could help more people.

When the judge left that night, I had some hope that maybe life would get a little better, and I thanked God. I had more to be grateful for than I realized then. The judge's next stop was to meet with people who owned our apartments and with people representing the community organization in our neighborhood.

One of those people said, "It is our understanding that people from that culture often get rid of Ebola contamination by burning down the places where sick people live."

So the judge said, "I want you to spread the word that if anyone does anything that harms or frightens this family— anything from setting a fire to spray painting their door with insults—that I will classify that action as a hate crime. And I will make sure they are prosecuted."

Early in the week, Presbyterian Hospital said that the emergency room doctor who first saw Eric didn't know that he was from West Africa because the computer system didn't send the doctor all the information. But on Friday, Presbyterian Hospital admitted that no computer glitch happened. The emergency room doctor didn't notice what was on the records.

The last time I spoke to Eric was on Friday. After the phone was ringing for a long time, he picked it up. I said hello, and I heard some sounds coming from the phone, like Eric was trying to talk: a gurgling sound, as if he were choking on something in his throat. I knew they'd put a tube down his throat and he could not talk. That was the last time I reached him on the phone. I called other times, but either the operator wouldn't put me through or no one

answered in his room. I was completely cut off from knowing about Eric. No one from the hospital called me.

At noon, a woman from the Health Department told the
media who were all waiting outside in the parking lot that
we were being moved to another place. The county would
soon have a place for us to live, she said.

"Will we know where that place is?" the reporters said.

"No. We will not disclose the location," she said. "The
move will be very soon." We were expecting the judge to
arrive, but he didn't.

He was still trying to find a place for us. The judge was
calling everywhere, but no one would agree. His office
called the Greater Dallas Apartment Association and the
Dallas Housing Authority. They said no. His office called
more places. And more. They all said no. We could not live
in their places.

Then the judge talked to Dallas mayor Mike Rawlings.
Mayor Rawlings used to be the head of a big Dallas ad
agency called TracyLocke. Then he was CEO of Pizza Hut.
The pizza restaurant then was named one of the best places
to work in Dallas. Before he was mayor, Mike Rawlings was
helping the homeless and got money to build a big homeless shelter. People called him the Homeless Czar.

When he was thinking about running for mayor of Dallas, his son asked him, "What would the virtuous man do?"
And so he ran for mayor.

The mayor knew so many people. He thought he would
so easily find us a place to live. But everyone was turning
him down, too. After some hours, he came back to the
judge and said, "We'll put them in my son's house."

The judge fist-bumped the mayor on the chest with both
his fists and said, "Now that's what I call leadership. Let's

get them over there." The mayor's son had bought a little house in a part of Dallas called Oak Cliff and was having it painted and all fixed up.

"We will put the Troh family in the front of the house," the mayor said. His wife and his son were concerned at this idea.

But the mayor told them, "There is no other place. We have to get Louise and her family out of the apartment." He and the judge were telling the reporters that having us stay with things Eric had touched was not sanitary—a health hazard.

So the mayor's wife and son said okay. They brought in some beds for us to sleep in. The judge drove over to the house to make sure that he could find it and have a nearby place to park where we could all run into the house if the reporters were following.

One more step was needed before we could move. We had signed that we would obey the order to stay in the apartment and not leave at all for twenty-one days. So the judge had to get a new order allowing us to move to a new living place where we would stay for the rest of our quarantine. When that was ready, he headed to our apartment to pick us up. The judge's people had been calling churches to see if someone would help us. Nobody called Wilshire. But when they called the Catholics, the judge used words from the Bible.

"What I told them is there is literally no more room at the inn, and I need your help," he told the reporters later. So while the mayor was moving beds into his son's house, people at the Catholic diocese were asking the Dallas bishop, Kevin Farrell, if he would let our family stay at a Catholic retreat center.

The bishop called the mayor and told him to bring us over. "When I got the call from the bishop, it really was a gift from God," the mayor said on television. On that day it was all secret. No one was allowed to know where we were going. We didn't know ourselves. Even the judge didn't know that the place had been changed from the mayor's son's house.

But before the judge could get back, the cleanup team arrived at our apartment. Whenever the Health Department workers came to take our temperatures, they wore regular clothes. They came inside the apartment and stood by us every day. Sonya said they were going by the science, which said Ebola isn't highly contagious and could not be passed through the air like flu or colds, and they would not give in to fear. But the cleanup workers came in yellow plastic suits with gas masks and big gloves. We couldn't see their faces. Their shoes were covered. They looked like spacemen. They were covered in plastic, and they put plastic everywhere.

It was so frightening: so much plastic to keep the virus out and to keep the virus in. We had been living in that apartment with Eric for almost a week and also living there after he went to the hospital. We had no plastic to protect us. But, oh yes, we were infected, too. So they needed plastic between them and us.

I said, "Why are you doing this?"

They took Eric from here six days earlier. They were just making the public afraid. They made it look like this place was all infected. They brought five, six, seven big trucks and fire trucks. They put fear in the people. People called to tell me they'd sealed off my car with black plastic that they taped all around it.

"That car has been out there in the hot sun for days," I said. "What could be in it now?" But they sealed it anyway.

When I saw how they were making everyone so scared, I was even more afraid that someone might do something to us. "Let's pray that God lets us stay alive," I told my nephews.

We weren't allowed to leave while the cleanup men tore off the sheets and pillows. They took all the towels and washcloths. I had already washed all these things. I had Cloroxed them. All the clothes Eric had worn were in a sealed bag, I told them.

"You don't need to be doing this."

But they didn't listen.

They put the bag of Eric's clothes into a barrel and started throwing all my clothes into the barrels. They were just dumping things, tearing up everything, slashing the bed and breaking things so that they fit into the barrels. They sawed my fifty-five-inch television in half. It was a Samsung television, a real good one. My daughter saved up to buy me that television as a present.

I know they were just doing what they had been hired to do, but my heart was breaking as I watched them throw out all my pretty African clothes that are so expensive and that I will never be able to replace, like the suit my friend sent me that cost $150. I had paid her only $120 so far. All our shoes, our hairbrushes, my jewelry, the gold chain that is the only thing I have from my daughter Kebeh, Karsiah's trophies from football, the letters from colleges recruiting him, the boys' clothes, the coats they need for winter, Karsiah's clothes, Oliver's, Jeffrey's.

Timothy lost his school uniforms, and all his shoes that he loved so much. Some of these shoes cost $150 a pair. I saved so hard to buy them. They took his basketball and his football.

"How am I ever going to go to school?" Timothy asked me, looking like he might cry. I didn't know what to tell him.

All the things I had worked so hard to buy, everything that made up my life: the men in yellow suits destroyed things Eric had never even seen or been near. I showed them his suitcase. It was zipped up. Nothing could get out. But they took all the luggage and threw it in the barrels.

"Eric wasn't even in these rooms or these closets," I told them.

People from Liberia had sent me T-shirts from the memorial service for my daughter Kebeh. I was saving them. They dug those shirts out from a drawer where they were deep down under other clothes. They wouldn't listen to anything I said. They threw away pots and pans, broke dishes and glasses.

I stopped trying to talk to them. They would not listen. We stood back then, making ourselves smaller and smaller, just watching our lives be slashed and broken. The cleanup men were working so hard that one of them started feeling sick, like he was about to faint. He went outside to rest and open up his mask. After that they didn't move so fast.

Did they have to destroy everything we had? Later, when the two nurses who cared for Eric had Ebola, they didn't destroy everything in their homes. They said it was because the nurses went to the hospital right away when they knew they were sick and didn't stay as long at home. But they didn't destroy all the equipment at the hospital, either; they decontaminated it. I'd already decontaminated my apartment. I told them, but nobody would believe me.

The judge was ready to take us to our new place, but he did not want the reporters following us. Helicopters were flying everywhere, all around our apartment. Judge Jenkins worked for the Obama election, and he knows people in the White House. So he called the White House to ask if they would make the helicopters stop flying.

"You want us to put a no-fly zone over an apartment in Dallas?" said this person the judge won't name, but many say was the president himself.

"Yes," the judge said.

"I don't believe we will be able to do that," the White House person said.

So the judge came to take us away. The health workers told me that I could take a purse with me. I put some clean underwear in my purse so I'd have something to change into. But now they said, "No purse." They let me take one car key and two bottles of vitamins sealed in ziplock bags. That's all. We were allowed to walk out in our clothes and nothing else.

The worst was losing the gold chain from Kebeh, my daughter who died. But all our papers were gone, too, and so were all our pictures: all taken from us. They told me that they put our passports, some family pictures, and my Bible in a barrel and that I would get them back sometime. Later I heard that they filled 155 barrels from my little apartment. They worked for four days tearing up the carpet and spraying the walls. They took all those barrels and burned them. All I ever got back were some documents and my Bible. Everything else was gone forever.

When the judge came to lead us out of the door, he was wearing a blue shirt and khakis: no mask, no gloves, no yellow suit. He said he didn't want us to feel that we were all alone, the only humans, with people who looked like spacemen all around us. As we left, the news reporters started taking pictures of us. The boys put their heads down so that their faces wouldn't show so much. I didn't look at the cameras. We looked so little, like people running away. All the news media people were following. Pastor George saw us on television that night and he thought, *I have to go and help Louise.*

The judge put us in his white Ford Explorer, now surrounded by police cars. The police stayed in front and back and on the sides of us. I think the police cars tried to block the reporters from following. Then all the helicopters disappeared. Later, when the judge called his friend at the White House, he told him that the helicopters disappeared.

"I'm sorry we weren't able to help you with that," the man said. "I'm glad it went well."

The judge and his staff wanted so much to keep where we were going secret that they planned to take us in one car to a big garage and then switch us to another car and drive out another way so that the reporters would not know we were in a different car. But then the judge decided that was not such a good plan. He would just drive us and see what happened.

This car ride that lasted maybe twenty minutes became famous, which wasn't good for the judge at all. People said he should not have allowed us in his car. The next day, one hundred children at his daughter's elementary school stayed home. People picketed the school. A woman called his nine-year-old little girl disgusting. When his wife showed up to serve lunch at the school, they weren't going to let her around the food at first. A man filed a complaint with Texas Child Protective Services against the judge. The man who filed told the reporter that he believed the judge was endangering his child and could be endangering other students at her school.

In the *Dallas Morning News,* a man named Mike Jenkins, not related to the judge, wrote that the judge "appears to wear 'compassion' on his sleeve for the express purpose of self-aggrandizement, as if to say, 'Here I am to save the day.'"

He continued, "The proper role of a Chief Emergency Response officer is to stay out of the way of the proper responders. . . . I can think of no reason why he should have gone into the apartment that Thomas Eric Duncan was staying in before he went to the hospital or a reason for him to personally drive the family to isolation."

"I believe this was all for show—plain and simple." This man wrote that the judge was only thinking about reelection, which was coming up in November.

But the judge responded to critics like this man by saying, "These are people who should be treated with dignity. They are my constituents, too."

In the judge's car, I was in the front and the boys were in the back. When we passed through the gates of the apartment, it seemed as if we were getting out of prison. To be outside going down a road was so good. But we were going to another place where we could be confined.

The judge asked us what we needed. Timothy said he needed a basketball. The judge promised to get him one.

Oliver said, "Why do so many people hate us?"

"People don't hate you. They were just afraid," the judge said. "People who are afraid look for a bad guy. They want someone to blame so they won't be so afraid. But you are not the bad guys."

"People didn't act like this when Kent Brantly came home," Oliver said, talking about the American doctor who went to Liberia for the Christian charity Samaritan's Purse, got Ebola, and was brought back to the United States.

"No. They sure didn't," the judge said.

When we drove away, some reporters in cars were still following us. When the judge was a student at Baylor University, he was arrested once for a car chase with Baylor security and Waco police. So maybe he was remembering those days. Once he went so fast across a highway with cars coming everywhere that I yelled out, "Oh, God. I am going to die right now."

He drove around corners and under bridges and down little streets. The judge twisted and turned down street after street. The boys in the back were squealing and I shut my eyes. But he lost them. We were only about fifteen miles from our apartment, but it seemed like a long way.

We were in a part of Dallas called Oak Cliff where I never go. There are too many highways between our neighborhood and Oak Cliff. I don't like to drive on highways. I felt like I was going to a country far away. On the way to Oak Cliff, the judge got a call saying that the Catholics were going to have us live at the retreat center, and so we weren't going to the mayor's son's house. The judge got the address for the center on his GPS: 901 Madison Avenue. But the GPS took us to 901 South Madison Avenue.

We parked in front of a deserted house that was falling down with bushes all grown up around it and a tree growing out of the porch. I knew that house would be full of snakes.

"Oh, Jesus," I said. "This is where you want us to live? This is how you treat us like one of your own? I am not getting out. You can just take us back to our apartment because we will not stay here."

"It must be a mistake," the judge said. He got out of the car and started walking around. The only people with us were in the sheriff's cars.

One of them must have seen what was wrong because the judge came back to the car and said, "Don't worry. We're at the wrong place." We were at 901 South Madison Avenue. We were supposed to be at 901 North Madison Avenue. We turned the car around and drove a few blocks in the other direction.

When we came to a driveway with a gate and a high wire fence around a big piece of land, he turned in. There was a sign with English and Spanish on it that said, "Catholic Conference and Formation Center." We passed a long building and went through a parking lot, past a seating area with benches and a cross in it, and past a maintenance garage with pickups parked outside. Nice little brick houses were set in a large field with space between them.

We drove past five or six sheriff's cars facing different directions. Some were facing so they could watch the gate, some facing the house we would live in, others just sitting around in other places so the deputies could watch the grounds.

The judge kept driving until he came to a house in the very back that had the words "Casa 7" on it. "Here we are," he said. A mat on the porch had pictures of a ladybug and a butterfly and the word "Welcome."

It was so beautiful, the trees around, everything clean and the fence that no one could get into. This house had four bedrooms and two baths, and a big kitchen with white cabinets and white counters with lots of room for cooking. Light came into the living room and kitchen. The bedrooms were darker, with not so many windows and coverings on them. Darkness might help us feel safe.

All the events were canceled for the time we were there. No one was around. We would be safe here, the judge said. There was no TV in the house, but later the county brought a TV. I did not want to watch it. The news was too terrible.

The mayor of Dallas was there to say welcome and tell us we would be safe. People said he shouldn't have come around us. Later that week, a lady who works for him came to his house wearing a mask. She knew he had visited us.

He asked her, "Are you wearing that now when you visit patients?"

And she said, "Just at your house."

Everyone treated us like we were poison that would kill them if they even came around anyone who had seen us. When the judge and the mayor left, I let the boys choose their rooms. Each bedroom had twin beds in it. Everything was so quiet. No traffic. No people.

So I went to my room and sat on the flowered bedspread. I was crying and so afraid of what had been on the news. The president of Liberia, Ellen Johnson Sirleaf, said that Eric knew he had Ebola, and he should be punished for bringing it to America. She was not even thinking about this very sick man who did nothing wrong. I was angry at her and I'm still angry at her. She never showed any concern or love for him. She just sold him to the Americans. Is that how she treats her people?

She could have said, "Would you please help him?" Why would she just jump to conclusions instead? She never cared about his life. What if it had been her own son? Would she say that?

The Dallas district attorney also said that he might press criminal charges against Eric for bringing Ebola. He said maybe Eric could be charged with aggravated assault using a deadly weapon, for having "exposed the public to a deadly virus knowingly, which would be criminal intent."

Eric might be put in prison for twenty years. These words made me so afraid. If Eric got well, he could be punished with prison. I had not forgotten that Eric failed to tell me about the pregnant girl who later died of Ebola; I could not forgive this deception. But I do not believe that he knew he had gotten Ebola from that girl. No one had died of it in his village then. He had no symptoms. I could not believe that he would risk infecting us all in Dallas.

This man was a sick person, suffering, crying in pain, but people were treating Eric like he *was* Ebola, a virus instead of a person who had done nothing to deserve this disease. I heard that some Liberians were wearing T-shirts that said, "Liberians are people. Not a virus." People were not remembering that about Eric. They were being so careless about his life.

I was just praying and praying for God to help us. I was thinking that the world is watching America. Eric was a young man; they weren't going to let him die. But if he doesn't die, he might go to prison. I was thinking that I had done the wrong thing in having him come to America. If he had stayed in Liberia, he might have been better off. I cried and cried.

Everything I owned was destroyed. I could never go back to my home. I might die. My loved ones might die. I was in prison in this place with a fence and sheriff's cars sitting

outside. No car. No job. If I tried to leave, I would be arrested. And where would I go? Who would hide us? I went
down on my knees and prayed that God would help. Only
God could help.

There was a Bible in the room and I wanted to open it to
read Psalm 121. But the Bible opened to Psalm 116. Here
is some of what I read:

> I love the Lord, for he heard my voice;
> he heard my cry for mercy.
>
> Because he turned his ear to me,
> I will call on him as long as I live.
>
> The cords of death entangled me,
> the anguish of the grave came over me;
> I was overcome by distress and sorrow.
>
> Then I called on the name of the Lord:
> "Lord, save me!"
>
> The Lord is gracious and righteous;
> our God is full of compassion.
>
> The Lord protects the unwary;
> when I was brought low, he saved me.
>
> Return to your rest, my soul,
> for the Lord has been good to you.
>
> For you, Lord, have delivered me from death,
> my eyes from tears,
> my feet from stumbling,

that I may walk before the Lord
in the land of the living.

I trusted in the Lord when I said,
"I am greatly afflicted";

in my alarm I said,
"Everyone is a liar."

What shall I return to the Lord
for all his goodness to me?

I will lift up the cup of salvation
and call on the name of the Lord.

I will fulfill my vows to the Lord
in the presence of all his people.

Precious in the sight of the Lord
is the death of his faithful servants.

Truly I am your servant, Lord;
I serve you just as my mother did;
you have freed me from my chains.

I will sacrifice a thank offering to you
and call on the name of the Lord.

I will fulfill my vows to the Lord
in the presence of all his people,

in the courts of the house of the Lord—
in your midst, Jerusalem.
Praise the Lord.

When I read those words, I felt God was with me. I made a vow then that if I did not die, if I got out of this terrible situation, I would try to make money so that I could help people of Liberia. I would build a church in Liberia. I would try to help orphans, maybe build an orphanage for them. And I would also give money to Wilshire.

Then I was calm and finally I could sleep.

# "You Have Lost the Man"

Being in a secret place made us feel safer but also so much more alone. Having hundreds of reporters outside the door was scary. Now only the sheriffs were outside. The sheriff's deputies were maybe to protect me, maybe to arrest me. Hardly anyone even knew where we were. It was like disappearing from the earth but still having voices follow you everywhere. One day I was just an ordinary woman, going to work every day. Now people were always ringing, ringing, ringing. I had no one to help me understand what was happening.

Then Jesse Jackson called.

"Louise, I want to come and see you," he said. "I will help you."

"I'm in quarantine," I said.

"I don't care. I will get them to let me see you," he said.

So I told him to come, and I also gave him the number of Eric's family in North Carolina.

I missed my old life so much. Sonya from the Health Department and Judge Jenkins were being friends, but they were not people I knew from before. So I was surprised and so happy when Pastor George came to visit on Saturday afternoon. After seeing us on television, he knew he wanted to come be with us.

When the judge heard that George Mason was my pastor, he told him, "We need to get you over there." So they met and drove over, but no one told me he was coming.

"I am so happy to see you, Pastor," I said. "Come, Timothy, meet Pastor George." He didn't know Timothy or Oliver or Jeffrey. None of them had gone with me to church. Only the women and children in our family had gone.

It was kind of awkward to meet new people because nobody could come close or shake hands. We could only stand there and look at each other. Pastor George said later that we all looked dazed, confused about everything, like refugees coming from a war.

The judge had been on the phone all the way over to our house, and he was still talking when he came in. He got off the phone finally and said CNN had found out where we were. He didn't want them to put the address on the air.

This mystery of where we were was all over the news. One guy on the Internet said he knew that we were in a house in Richardson, northeast of Dallas. He was going by to see if he could spot us. Other people started driving by that house. But we were not there. We were far across the city.

If people knew we were in Oak Cliff, maybe the neighbors would complain. The bishop might get angry phone calls. The news media might start trying to climb the fences. Or even worse, people might try to harm us. So many sheriff's deputies were around the house not only to keep us inside, but to make sure no one came to harm us.

The judge was making a deal with CNN. If I would talk with Anderson Cooper again, they would not say where I was or send reporters and cameras to the gate. I would just answer some questions on the phone. So I did.

This time Anderson said something about the president of Liberia's terrible statements: that Eric came to America when he knew he had Ebola. She was wrong to accuse him without knowing the facts. But this president was being so eager to please America that I was worrying about what she might do. I have sons in Liberia still.

"I have three boys over there," I said to Anderson. "They better not go after my family." There was so much to worry me. My children in America were in danger of having Ebola and my sons in Africa were in danger of being blamed for things they knew nothing about. But mostly I thought all the time about Eric. I could remember his sweetness so well. So I gave Anderson Cooper a message.

"I'm asking the American government. The same medicine you gave to the people who came from Liberia, please give Eric Duncan. He is a young man. You can save his life."

Anderson Cooper put exactly what I said on the television. I liked Anderson for that, but I did not want to talk with the reporters anymore. So many had my telephone number. They were asking me the same questions over and over. So I asked Pastor George if he would talk to them for me. "I can do that if you give me permission," he said. "I have to keep what you tell me confidential unless you say I can talk about it."

"Yes, you can," I said.

So every time after that, Pastor George would tell them, "Louise has told me to say." That Sunday, television reporters from all over the world were in the church at Wilshire.

They knew that I didn't want to talk, but some of them still called me.

The media said Eric was doing well early on that Saturday. He was recovering. I was jubilant, so happy, but not too surprised. When the two American doctors had been flown in from Africa with Ebola and recovered, I thought Eric would, too. But there was some trouble. They said the drug they gave the doctors, ZMapp, had been all used up. So they put Eric on an experimental drug called brincidofovir, an antiviral.

They said they also couldn't give Eric the doctor Kent Brantly's blood, which could help him, because it was the wrong type.

Since then I have wondered, why couldn't they get some blood from Africa? Lots of people there have Ebola. This was just one of the questions I started to ask myself. Other friends and family members who live in other parts of the country were calling to ask me questions also. The questions and strange stories multiplied. A person who does cleaning at the hospital told that when they went in to clean Eric's room there was blood everywhere: on the floor, the ceilings, the walls. She said it looked like wild animals had been fighting in that room. What could that mean? I didn't know, but it hurt my heart to hear such things.

Eric's mother told me that when she talked to him he told her he was so alone and in the dark. No one came to see him. They just left him alone all the time, he said.

I remembered then that on Thursday when he told me that people were coming into the room, he sounded nervous, maybe scared, "They are coming. They are coming. I have to go," he said.

Another woman who worked at the hospital had been saying that Eric was moved to a room where people did not recover. She saw no doctors going in and out of there.

These scary stories tormented me. I had no information from the hospital. I am alone and the only people calling me have stories from everywhere—rumors, lies, maybe. But what is the truth? Eric's picture wearing a green shirt was everywhere on the news. But there were no pictures of Eric in the hospital, and none of the people who loved him were able to see him.

I heard that hospital records said he was up and walking around during the first part of his stay. They said he drank some Sprite and watched a movie. But when I talked to Eric on the phone Monday, he told me he couldn't walk around because of all the machines. When I saw him on Monday after work, he was too weak to even sit up.

Stanley Gaye, president of the Liberian Community Association of Dallas/Fort Worth, kept calling me every day, sometimes many times a day, saying, "Are you all right? Are you in pain?"

When Stanley called later on that Saturday, he did not start in the usual way.

"I heard the news. Bad news," he said.

"What news? That my husband is dead? I have not heard that."

"Disregard," he said. "This must be a false report."

"No one has told me this."

"Well then, it is not true."

At that time, I did not believe Eric was dead. I called the hospital again, but I was not able to talk with him.

Later that Saturday, a friend called to tell Youngor that

Eric had died. Youngor does not know where she got that information: maybe the Internet. Then a woman who said she worked for Presbyterian called.

"I'm so sorry about your loss," she said.

"My daddy is dead?" Youngor said in a scared voice. She started crying and the woman said, "Oh, I'm sorry that is a mistake. It was not true." The lady hung up.

Later she called back and said, "I am calling to talk to you about the hospital bill." Youngor was confused. The woman went on to say that the bill for Eric's treatment would be about $1 million. The woman asked, would Youngor and her family be able to pay?

"We're not talking about the bill. First save his life and then we will talk about the bill," Youngor said. "We will find a way to pay. We will all work to pay off that bill. Don't worry."

But the strangeness was only starting.

At 10:00 that night a friend of mine in another state called to say that she saw on the Internet that Eric was dead. I know that many things on the Internet are not true. But sometimes the things that people put on there are the true things that the people with power don't want other people to know. I was thinking that he might have died, but I wasn't sure because this didn't seem like proof.

I called the hospital. They said they would put me through to his room. The phone rang and rang but no one answered.

So I went to sleep. My niece called at 1:00 a.m. on Sunday. She was crying bitterly.

"You have lost the man," she said. "You have lost the man."

"Where did you hear this?" I asked.

"I saw it on *ABC News*."

I started crying then and everyone woke up and started crying, too. Oliver was crying and banging on things. We were all in my room crying and feeling terrible for about four hours until we were so worn out that I said we must go back to our beds to sleep.

That night in the single bed in my bedroom, I felt Eric's spirit come into the room. I could feel it go behind me, between me and the wall behind the bed. I felt him in my spirit. He was leaving this earth. He called my name twice. Later, my son in Africa called to say that he, too, had felt Eric in his spirit and believed he was dead.

Sunday morning, I called Karsiah. "I believe your father is dead," I told him.

He started to cry.

"Don't get sick with crying. I'm the one supposed to be crying," I said.

Pastor George came later in the day on Sunday, and he saw that we were all just grieving so much.

"No," he said. "Eric is still alive. I would have heard if he was dead. The report was wrong. They made a mistake." The reporters were calling and saying that the report had been a mistake. The television was saying that he was still alive. I wanted to think that he was living and would get well. So then we tried to believe that Eric was still alive.

I called the hospital again. They said I couldn't talk to him because doctors were in his room. I called again. They said tests were being done on him, call later. Finally, they said they would ring his room but again the phone rang and rang and no one answered.

Pastor George said the church was going to have a prayer vigil on Wednesday for Eric and my family. He said Liberian pastors would speak and everyone would pray to God that he would get well and that no one else would get Ebola. People from all over Dallas would be there.

When he talked to me of this vigil, I thought he said that he was planning a memorial service and he wanted to know if we wanted to have it in the church or at the house we were in. I wondered why he was talking about a memorial service if Eric wasn't dead. It seemed strange to me.

Pastor George did not like that he wasn't allowed to hug us. He is not usually just standing far from people without touching.

"We have to find some way to show the love," he said. Then he crossed his arms over his chest so they were like an "X" and he patted his hands on his chest. "How's that? We can do that for a hug." So now when we saw each other and before Pastor George left we would do this hugging motion.

On Monday, Eric's nephew Josephus Weeks, who has been in America many years and served in the Iraq war, drove from North Carolina with Eric's mother, Nowai, and his sister Mai. Eric was the youngest of Nowai's seven children.

Mai, a nurse and Josephus's mother, is the one my daughter Youngor called before she dialed 911 to take Eric to the hospital. When Eric got to the hospital, he put me as the next of kin and person to contact, but Mai begged me to put her on the hospital list. And I did.

When I went into quarantine, I lost all chance to find out what was really happening with Eric. If I called the hospital, the doctors would not talk to me. Maybe they took me off the list. Now Mai and her son Josephus were the people the doctors talked to. Karsiah was in school so many miles away, without a car to get him to Dallas. So I gave him any news of his father.

By now Josephus had talked with Jesse Jackson, and they had arranged for him to come to Dallas on Tuesday. I never heard from Jesse Jackson again.

When the family got to town on Monday, they went to the hospital to see Eric. The hospital would not let them into Eric's room. Eric's sister Mai offered to put on a suit like the other nurses. But they said no. His sister tried to leave a phone for Eric, but again the hospital said no.

They said Eric's relatives could see him on a video camera that was set up in the room. On the little screen, they saw that Eric was in bed. The picture did not show the monitors all around him monitoring his condition. Why did it not show the monitors that would have proved he was alive? The picture just showed part of him lying in the bed. You could see his body under the sheet and his head. His face was facing up and not clear—all fuzzy. You could see some white from his eyes, which were bulging out of his head.

My new friend from Washington, DC, Saymendy Lloyd, was in town with Eric's family and sent me a picture of the video. Karsiah got one, too, on his iPhone. Along with the photo, she texted me, "Your husband is not looking good at all. You better get his son down here to see him."

Karsiah had stayed at school working on his studies. But on Tuesday he came to Dallas. He went to the hospital and told them that he was Eric's son. They were going to let him in to see Eric, but then a doctor came up and said Karsiah wasn't on the list of relatives. Only Josephus and Eric's sister were on the list, even though Karsiah was the closest relative.

It was wrong, but Karsiah was turned away. He never got to see his father. He planned to go back the next morning and try to get in again, but by then it was too late.

Before Karsiah arrived on Tuesday, the Reverend Jesse Jackson came to town. He went with Eric's family to see the monitor of Eric again. When Eric's mother saw her son like that, she cried and lost all her strength. She couldn't look anymore. Jesse Jackson had to help her away.

Then the family and Jesse Jackson met with the doctors. The communications director of the Liberian Community Association of Dallas/Fort Worth, Alben Tarty, was there and he told me what happened.

Eric's mother said, "I want to see my son's whole body. He is not even shaking. I want to touch my son."

Jesse Jackson said maybe that wouldn't be possible, but he asked the doctors if they could put her in a room with glass between her and him where she could see his whole body. The doctors said they could not.

Then Alben said that Eric's mother said, "People in Liberia are surviving Ebola. Please tell me why my son is not getting well."

The doctors said, "His vital signs are good. His diarrhea is improving."

So Alben said, "All the things you said are giving the impression that Duncan's health has improved. Can we confidently say Duncan is improving?"

They said, "We can't say for sure because every day it changes. We can't really say what will happen tomorrow."

When Alben told me this story, he said, "Everything the doctors said was about that man's health. But that man was already dead."

Eric's mother called me later and she believed the same.

Before Jesse Jackson left, he held a press conference to talk about Eric. "He got sick, went to the hospital," Jesse Jackson said. "He didn't have insurance . . . , and they turned him away. So they sent him back into the community with a contagious disease, and for that there must be some liability."

Then Jesse Jackson talked about the medicine.

"They are saying no more doses [of ZMapp]," Jackson said. "That seems strange to only have enough medicine for two patients in the whole country.

"It seems the way we treated the Americans in Georgia and Nebraska is different than the way we treated a victim here in Dallas," Jackson said, meaning two white doctors who came back from Liberia and were sent to hospitals with specialized treatment facilities in Georgia and Nebraska.

The hospital put out its own statement that ran in newspapers: "Thomas Eric Duncan was treated the way any other patient would have been treated, regardless of nationality or ability to pay for care. We have a long history of treating a multi-cultural community in this area."

Later, Eric's mother called me. "He didn't move at all," she said. "He wasn't alive. If he was alive he would have moved. Eric never moved." She was already mourning her son because she believed that he was dead.

Karsiah thought so, too. So did Alben. Pastor George said they were wrong. What should I believe? It was on the news that since they had the first Ebola case, they had learned from this first man, now they know what to do. What did that mean? I was getting so suspicious. All I heard were rumors and news accounts that are not the same. No one from the hospital talked to me. I heard only gossip and speculation.

With so many people saying Eric was dead, I could not eat anything. On Tuesday night, I ate some rice, thinking that I needed some strength for the next days. On Wednesday, I was cooking when a knock on the door came at about 9:00 a.m.

I went to my room to get a bit straightened up. Oliver answered the door.

"Hey, man. Give me some love," he said to Pastor George. They both did the hugging sign. Judge Jenkins was with Pastor George and the judge was carrying his Bible. Pastor George had given his Bible to Timothy. So he didn't have one with him.

"Why are you here so early?" I said, smiling.

They didn't really answer.

We called the boys from their rooms. The living room had three chairs with striped covers and wooden arms. The sofa was brown with wooden arms. It wasn't big enough for two people to sit on when they had to make sure they weren't touching. So I sat in one chair and Timothy and Jeffrey sat in others. Oliver was on the sofa. The sun was coming in the sliding glass door. We had put a white bedsheet over it for a curtain. It was a sunny, warm day. The carpet was a pretty blue with green—cheerful.

Judge Jenkins and Pastor George stood in the middle of the room with their backs to the kitchen. We were all looking up at them. They had something to tell us, I could see that. But they weren't talking. The judge was holding his phone. He kept glancing at it.

"How are you doing?" Pastor George said.

"We are fine," I said.

Then we talked a little about movies the boys were watching or music. Something that wasn't important. The men were standing like they didn't know what to do. Putting their hands behind them, and then in their pockets. This was the way for five or ten minutes, with everyone just looking at each other.

When the judge's phone rang, he answered it.

"Okay," he said. "Thank you."

Then he put the phone in his pocket.

"Well, Louise, you may have been wondering why we came this morning. That was the hospital. I had to wait to hear from the hospital before I could tell you the news that Mr. Duncan passed this morning."

I cried out in pain and fell from my chair to the floor. I was curled into myself with my face on the rug. I turned away from the men. The pain in my body and spirit was so great that I could only cry out again and again. No words, just wailing from the pain of grief. I could not move from the floor, just sobbing and hurting.

I heard Oliver groan. His head was back on the sofa. He was staring at the ceiling, moaning. Jeffrey was quiet and very still.

We could not comfort each other because we were not allowed to touch, Judge Jenkins and Pastor George were not allowed to come closer than three feet. So they stood in the middle of the room. Pastor George had tears in his eyes. He moved closer to me so that he was almost above me. "Louise, oh, Louise, my dear, I am so sorry," he said.

"Am I going to die of Ebola?" Timothy said to the judge. My brave thirteen-year-old was finally breaking down. "Tell me now if I am going to die."

The judge crouched down like he was a baseball catcher with his arms open like he wanted Timothy to run toward him so that he could catch him and hold him. But we knew that couldn't happen.

"No, Timothy. You are not going to die. You are all right. We are doing all the things that will keep you safe."

"They couldn't save Eric because they got to him too late," Pastor George said. "That isn't going to happen to anyone here."

Eric died alone, surrounded by people in white suits and masks. No human was there to speak kindly to him. No one held his hand or calmed his fears.

Later we were told that his last words had been to a nurse who asked him what he wanted. Eric said, "I want to see my son."

"Where is your son?" she asked.

"He's at college where he's supposed to be," Eric said. He had come many thousands of miles hoping to meet his son, who loved him so much. But they never even saw each other. Why? I keep asking myself. Why didn't they let our son see his father? I think it might have been because he was already dead when they set up the picture phone call with his mother.

Another story was that Eric died with tears running down his face. He was not conscious, but the tears were real. That nurse, a man, said he told Eric that he was going to be all right and that he should just rest. The nurse said he got a tissue to wipe the tears away. Then about fifteen minutes later, Eric died. The nurse said he held Eric in his arms. He said he was so sad that Eric was all alone. The nurses said he was always so polite and grateful for everything they did. Eric was always that way.

On the day of the awful news, I could not stop crying until Timothy came to me and said, "Please don't cry, Mama. I want you to be with me. I want you to be happy." And so I worked to stop my crying.

After a while I was still. I got up from the floor. Karsiah was calling on the phone.

"Mama, I did not get to see my father. I don't know what happened," he said. "God is going reveal whatever they did to my father."

That day Karsiah also got a call from the president of Angelo State University. He thought the president was telling him not to come back to school for the rest of the semester. Later, the president said there was a misunderstanding and that he was just giving Karsiah the usual two weeks of school for bereavement. But Karsiah didn't think he had the right to come back to school, and he was very upset. When he told me, I asked Judge Jenkins what to do. Karsiah hadn't even been able to see his father. He had never been around anyone who had Ebola. The judge said the decision was unfair and that he would see to it.

We were all just sitting, feeling so confused and sad. "Something has to be done," Oliver said. "This is not right. They did not do that man right. We have to do something." He meant that the hospital was liable.

This talk about suing the hospital was going to grow in the next month. Lawyers would be calling more. It was just Oliver's bad luck to be with me when Eric came to Dallas. Now we were joined in grief. Maybe he thought I should be suing, or that Karsiah should be.

I felt the same way Oliver did about justice. Whoever sued had to have a legal right, and I might have some right because Liberian customary marriage law might consider us married. Karsiah and the three other children Eric had after Karsiah would have some rights. Two of those children were in Africa and one in North Carolina. Perhaps Eric's mother, who was in North Carolina, and his father, still in Africa, could sue. But I was not thinking about money or rights on that day. I was thinking only that if the hospital didn't treat Eric well, they had done wrong.

"We will hold them accountable," Pastor George said. "The judge and I are both committed to finding out the truth of what happened for you."

I knew the judge was a lawyer who helped people who had wrong done to them. Before he was the Dallas county judge, Judge Jenkins made a lot of money because he won so many cases. Winning against Presbyterian would not be easy, he said. I did not think that I wanted to sue anyone, but I also did not want to act like Eric's life was not important.

Then Pastor George said, "Louise, you have to decide whether you're going to take vengeance out of anger, or you're going to leave vengeance to God. God is not mocked. The truth will come out. If we judge them publicly before knowing all the facts, we will make it seem like we don't care about the truth. Jesus said the truth will set you free. So we must only say what we know to be true. We have a chance to be a witness for our faith in how we handle this."

I know he was right because that's what the Bible says, but this was a hard choice for me. I was so hurt and angry. I tried to get help for Eric but the hospital sent us away. I tried to see him but the hospital sent me away. I tried to talk with Eric but the hospital operators wouldn't connect me. So many strange things happened with no explanation.

Karsiah was already saying that he would let God be the judge. He is a godly boy. And then Pastor George asked me, "Would you like me to help you write a statement about how you feel?"

So Pastor George and I put out a statement that talked of our anger but not vengeance.

"I trust a thorough examination will take place regarding all aspects of his care. I am now dealing with the sorrow and anger that his son was not able to see his father before he died. This will take some time, but in the end, I believe in a merciful God," I said in the statement.

I asked people to keep my family in their prayers.

I said of Eric, "His suffering is over. My family is in deep sadness and grief, but we leave him in the hands of God. Our deepest sympathies go out to his father and family in Liberia and here in America. Eric was a wonderful man who showed compassion toward all. . . . This has dramatically changed our lives, and we will be grieving for a long time."

I put thanks in my statement for Dallas, my church, and the Liberian community. I thanked Mayor Rawlings, Judge Jenkins, and Pastor George for the love and support they had shown me and my family during this ordeal.

"Without their help, I can't imagine how we could have endured."

The prayer vigil at Wilshire turned into a memorial service for Eric. About two hundred people came. One of them was Bishop Nathan S. Kortu, a spiritual leader in the Dallas-area Liberian community and pastor of New Life Fellowship Church from a suburb called Euless.

"I pray for a remedy for this dreaded disease. Let it come to an end, Father God, we are tired as a nation," Pastor

Kortu prayed. "We are tired as a region of Africa. Father God, we come to tell you we can't take it no more. We call upon your name, Your faithful name, Mighty Jesus, [that] Your Spirit of comfort will rest upon these children."

Then Pastor Mason spoke: "Over the past week we have heard people over and over again who are worried," Pastor Mason said. "They are worried about this virus coming to our country, coming into our life. This is an unwelcome guest, let us be honest. No one wants this virus in our community, in our city, or in our world.

"But when something is here, we embrace it not because it is good—it is bad—but we seek to find what God might do that is good in us and through us because of it."

"Our love for Louise has made this suffering come to us," said Pastor George. "When you love someone, you are vulnerable to suffering, and you are open to joy. Love is the deepest reality of life, and so you feel it all.

"This service is intended to draw people together, to call one another to God who is judge of the living and the dead, and to lay each of our lives before the mercy of God. The world likes to divide people up in all sorts of ways. And it likes to say that differences mean otherness.

"We Christians have a different attitude about that. We look at 'difference' differently. We think of the oneness of our humanity as children of God, because God has made us all the same underneath, has loved us and died for us in Christ, and so our differences can be embraced, not run from.

"Every day we have a choice to make about how we will live. Are we going to move away from people, out of fear? Are we going to protect ourselves and live for ourselves, or are we going to move toward one another out of love, because we know that the end of the story is already promised? It ends well. So we can have courage, we can live with faith. This is what it means to say that at the heart of all things is love."

All that day and night the reporters kept calling, but when I answered all I could do was cry. My daughters called and we cried together. At the house in Oak Cliff, we were alone again. Taking our temperatures. Sleeping alone. Staying away from one another.

"Please, Auntie, don't come near us," Oliver said. "I'm afraid because you were with that man. So when I see you I'm so afraid of you. I'm afraid you are going to be the next one to die."

My nephews were still wearing gloves around the house and washing the cook spoon I'd used before they dipped their food out. They were still washing their own dishes and taking them to their bedrooms with them. But now they started leaving the living room when I came in. They would go to their bedrooms and only come back out when I was in my own bedroom.

This was so painful to me. But I understood their fear.

# CHAPTER THIRTEEN

# Twenty-One Days and Counting

On Thursday, October 9, we'd been quarantined for ten days. This day and the next four days were the time of most danger. If we didn't get sick, our risk would go down. If we did get sick we could be dead in a week. Twenty days ago, I was in my apartment waiting for Eric to walk through my door. I can see his big smile and how his eyes found me. Now he is dead and my family may also die. I am alone again. Much more alone.

Again I am grieving, now with much greater grief. At the time Eric came, I was mourning my Liberian daughter. Now I have Eric's death to add to my sorrow. I am afraid again. Before Eric came I was afraid that I was too old, that he would not love me, that my heart would be hurt again. Those fears seem so little now. Everything I own has been destroyed. I have no home. I may die with all of my family.

A friend called to tell me, "You should be at a hospital, not hiding out." She thinks I have the choice about where I go, what I do. I do not. I have no choice now. No freedom. Always I protested unfairness. I protected myself and those I love by protesting. But protests can't protect us now.

War took the life I made in Liberia. Disease took the life I made in America. In the Ivory Coast, people didn't like us, maybe. But nobody was so cruel to blame us in our troubles. Now people say we should be killed for our misfortune.

Again and again I say, "We did nothing wrong."

Judge Jenkins told the media, "I think the world of that family and how they are handling with dignity and grace the very understated and difficult circumstances."

Pastor George tells the media that we did nothing wrong. God knows we are telling the truth. On Oct 9, Anderson Cooper said of Eric, "He lost his life because he reached out in a human moment to help someone else."

Pastor George said to him, "We have to decide how we are going to tell people's stories. Not everyone is a villain or a victim. Sometimes there's enormous courage involved in these acts. And while a tragedy did occur, people often act in noble ways and sometimes it costs them their lives."

The boys and I will be so afraid until day fourteen. We are still required to take our temperatures two times a day. But we are so frightened during this critical time that we take our temperatures many times. Now in the morning and at night, the health workers come, or Oliver calls us into the living room. We don't talk during the time it takes to register.

Then each of us takes out the thermometer and looks to see what the reading is. We call it out and the Health Department worker writes it down. Or Oliver writes it down and gives it to the Health Department when they call. We can take our temperatures as often as we want to. We keep the thermometers in our bedrooms. We can stay in there and use them without the others knowing that we are so afraid.

Once Oliver ate a Hot Pocket before taking his temperature. The reading was over 100°. He panicked. "I'm going to die," he said. "I have Ebola. This is it. "

"No, you just ate a hot food," I said. "I drank a hot drink and my temperature went up. You will be all right. Wait and take it again."

Oliver is the most frightened. Every time he talks to Sonya from the Health Department, he tells her some new thing that is scaring him. "I have this terrible pain at the lower part of my brain." Or "I got up from my bed this morning and I felt so dizzy. Do I have Ebola?"

Every time, Sonya says the same thing, "Did you take your temperature? Is it normal? If it's normal, you are okay."

It is easy to think the way Oliver does. Ebola symptoms are so broad: headache, muscle and joint ache, tiredness, weakness, lack of appetite. When you start to look for these things, you find yourself feeling them a lot. Every pain in your stomach, you think it might be Ebola. You feel a little hot, you run to take your temperature.

Timothy was feeling sick. I knew he had allergies, but fear clutches over every little thing. When the Health Department delivered Claritin for him to take, he got better. I try to keep my fear to myself because it might frighten Timothy. He is so angry at having to be here. I apologize and apologize, but I can't make things better.

I was trying not to cry so much. If I cried, Timothy would come to me and say, "Mama, stop crying. I want you to be happy with me." Many friends and family members would call every day, and they were so scared that they would be crying. I would not.

"Don't make me cry," I told them. "If I cry my temperature goes up and I don't want that."

Stanley Gaye from the Liberian Association called one day to say, "I heard you on CNN. You really need food to eat."

I said, "We are hungry. They brought some canned food here, and we don't do canned food. I want real food." We had food from the Red Cross. The delivery people were afraid to bring it into the house but Jesse, a Catholic deacon and the manager of the retreat center, was not afraid. So he brought it. I was despairing about ever getting any of the food we liked to eat.

"Can the ladies cook some African food for you?" Stanley said.

"I like to cook for myself. If you just get uncooked food and you call, someone will come and get it from you." I knew that I could ask Sonya from the Health Department. She was my friend.

They brought food and food and food, and pots and pans: cassava leaf, potato leaf, palm butter, fever leaf, eggplant, fresh tomatoes, seasoning, pepper. They even brought a wrap to tie around yourself so you don't get your clothes dirty when you are cooking.

But I did not have any appetite. I cooked food, but when I put it in my mouth, it had no taste—like sawdust. From when Eric died until we left Oak Cliff, I lost about twenty-five pounds.

Sonya picked up the fresh food and brought it to us. When the charities brought us food or toiletries or cleaning supplies, they would leave them outside. No one wanted to come near us. Once when the shower broke, a man named Jesse came to try to fix it. Oliver had tried to fix it, and he was telling Jesse what he had done, but he was also being

considerate of him. When Jesse went into the little bathroom, Oliver stayed back in the hall so that they would not
have a chance of brushing against one another.

Forty-eight other people who came in contact with Eric
were in voluntary quarantine. They had to take their temperatures every day. Some were being told to stay home
from work, not to go shopping or into crowds. Here's how
Mayor Mike Rawlings described it: "They can walk their
dog. But they can't go to church. They can't go to schools.
They can't go to shopping centers."

Some were health workers, some were people I know.
Many called me to see if we were all right. Everyone in Dal-
las was more afraid because Eric died. If one of us gets sick,
I wondered what their fear would do.

One day, a friend of my play daughter Mimico called her
to say that she heard I was dead. So Mimico called me and
called me, but I did not answer. So then she started calling
my daughters, and she could not get any of them to answer.
She was so afraid all day.

Finally I answered. She was so happy to hear my live
voice, but she didn't want me to know people were saying I
was dead. So she just said really calmly, "How are you?"

I call Mimico my play daughter because we are so close.
When Mimico first came to America, I visited to welcome
her. When she had her baby, I helped her by coming over
to bathe the baby every day. Mimico was in voluntary quarantine because she was happy for Eric to be in Dallas and
she came to welcome him. Just once. But now people said
she is in danger.

When she was quarantined, she was so frightened for
herself and her baby that she was not eating at all. When she

went to work, all she did was drink coffee. One day when she came home, she felt so shaky and ill. She felt dizzy and her stomach hurt. She took her temperature. It was 100°. She got so scared that she called the Health Department to tell them she had Ebola.

The woman on the phone said, "What have you eaten today?"

"I can't eat. I am too nervous to eat. I only drink coffee," Mimico said.

The woman laughed. "Have some food and drink a lot of water," she said. "You will feel better. You don't have Ebola."

So Mimico's daughter made her some soup, and she was all right again.

My daughter Mawhen Jallah only came into the apartment once on Thursday before the first time Eric went to the hospital. She saw him lying on the mattress nearest the fireplace feeling tired. She didn't touch him. She went into the kitchen, opened the refrigerator, and said, "You need some food. I'll go by Fiesta and get you some groceries." The day after Eric died, Mawhen's friend who takes care of her baby called her at work.

"They say your mom's husband has Ebola," she said. Later she called again and said, "I don't want to take care of your baby anymore."

Mawhen was shaking and so scared. She went to get her baby. Later, she saw some friends outside a store leaving as she was going in. She called out her friend's name. Her friend started running toward her and then she stopped. She waved at Mawhen but didn't walk any closer.

For a few days, the health officials didn't allow Mawhen to go to Parkland Hospital where she works in the laundry.

Then for three days they made her check in to have her temperature taken three times a day. She would check into the nurses' station and go to a separate room where the nurse would give her a thermometer. Once when her asthma was acting up, her temperature was 99.4°. The nurse told her not to leave the room. She sat there for three hours. Then the CDC called back to say that was a normal temperature. So they let her go back to work.

No friends came to my daughters' or my nieces' apartments to visit. On the Internet, Youngor read that people were saying that if someone killed our whole family, nobody would catch Ebola. Even her friends writing on Facebook said that her mother had caused Dallas to be infected.

My daughter Nopie, who picked Eric up from the airport, saw that a man online said that I brought the Ebola man to kill us all. He cursed me and Youngor.

When Nopie defended us, he said that when she came out of quarantine, he was going to come to her house to curse her. But he never came. People were putting my daughters' addresses online and were coming by their houses to point and say, "That's where they live." Children would not play with our children.

One reporter came to Youngor's house and sat outside the door for hours, but she wouldn't answer the door. When Youngor ordered cable TV, the man came to install but was afraid to come in. So he left. Then another one came. They told him that they were in quarantine for Ebola but their temperatures were not high. So he came in, but he wouldn't touch anything. He would point and tell them what to do.

A lady was supposed to move into the apartment across the porch from Youngor's family, but when she found out who they were, she wouldn't. The apartment was vacant for a long time.

One reporter called me and said, "You need to talk to me so people will know what's happening. Judge Jenkins isn't going to help you. He's running for reelection and he's too busy."

Dallas had a power blackout in Youngor's neighborhood. It lasted four days. Another reporter called: "How does it feel to know that your daughter and all her family are without power and can't leave their apartment?"

"How would it feel to you if you knew that was happening and you were imprisoned and couldn't help?" I said.

The reporters were calling so much. "Hi, Louise," they would say, as if they knew me. "How are you doing?" But they didn't know me.

"We want to help you," they said.

"We want to tell your story," they said.

I did not trust these reporters, and I didn't want to talk to them. I wanted to go back to my old life when people didn't know about me, and I could go where I wanted to go. And no one hated me. I don't like talking with the reporters, so I told them to call Pastor George.

All that time only the health workers and two people came to see us, the judge and my pastor. They were not allowed to touch us. They were not supposed to sit down on the furniture. So most of the time they stood three feet from us like they are supposed to. But when the others left, Pastor George got a chair from the kitchen and sat in the living room with us.

Every day Pastor George came to see us.

"Don't you have a home to go to?" I said. "Aren't people in your family afraid that you are here all the time? Why are you here?"

"Oh, Louise," he said. "I just have to come here."

Stanley Gaye called me almost ten times a day: "Are you feeling pain?"

My son Karsiah also called. He worried that I would die.

"Did you ever kiss him?" he asked.

"Yes."

"In the mouth."

"No, not in the mouth." I kissed Eric on the outside of his mouth but not in the mouth. "What difference does it make? I slept with him. We were in bed when he called you on the phone on your birthday."

"Oh, Mama. I'm really worried," he said.

"Just give it to God," I said.

People at Wilshire Baptist Church were writing notes to me. Pastor George brought hundreds of them and I read them all.

One was my favorite. It's from a little girl who wrote, "I am praying for you. We all love you like God loves you."

Pastor George came in with gifts sometimes. He brought DVDs for the boys to watch. Timothy made a list of what he wanted, and Pastor George brought a lot of action movies and comedies that boys like. He also brought some music and headphones.

Jeffrey had a laptop computer and was on it most of the time. Oliver was listening to music on his headphones. Timothy was outside in the back on a concrete patio bouncing the basketball or inside bouncing it on the floor or the walls. He was so angry that we had to be there; all the time he was bouncing that ball.

"I am sorry, Timothy," I said. "There is nothing I can do."

He would not sleep all night. He would come into my room and keep me awake talking. Then he would go to other rooms, always roaming around until about 4:00 in the morning, when he would finally go to sleep. There was a basketball court in the retreat center, but the boys never went to it. To go, they would have had to walk by the sheriff's cars, and they were afraid.

We all stayed inside except when Timothy went to the backyard and paced on the patio, bouncing, bouncing, and bouncing back and forth like a tiger with a ball. We are afraid to go out even in the front of the house. The longer we stayed in the house hidden, the more afraid of the world I was.

Days ten through fourteen we just survived. If you feel a pain in your stomach, you think maybe that's it. You feel a little hot, you think maybe it's the virus. Very, very scary. I was praying, "Please, God, I am innocent. I brought Eric here with a good mind so we could live our life together. Father, please."

I kept praying and praying. "Father, can you give me a second time to live so I can worship you. Please, Father, give me a second chance."

I spent some of my time cooking. Most of the time I was in my room in the back of the house praying or crying. I was always thinking about those dark nights Eric had in Presbyterian Hospital with no one. Nobody came to see him, he said, nobody was walking around. People called to tell us that he cried and cried, saying how much he loves his country and how he wishes he was there. Maybe it would have been better if he had never come to America.

Eric had no good life. He wanted all his life to come to America. He wanted only to work and help his family. To every one of us, he said, "When I have a job, I will do for you." To his father in Africa, "Be patient. I will send you money." To Timothy, "I will buy you shoes." To me, "You are the woman. I will give you the money to manage."

We both suffered. We asked for a little happiness. Why this terrible punishment? Why this terrible death, this fear, this time of terrible reputation? I do not blame God. I would never do that. But I think again and again about the hospital. Why did they treat this man the way they did?

After Eric passed away, I dreamed how he was sick in the hospital. He came into the house and lay down on the single bed in my room. He rolled and fell on the floor.

I said, "Why do you have to lie on the floor?"

His hair was covered in something white.

"Your hair is dirty," I said.

He wrapped himself with a sheet.

"Why are you lying down like this?" I said. But he didn't answer me. He just kept whimpering.

In the night sometimes, thinking I only have these twenty-one days to live, I am in the bed in the dark remembering Eric walking, turning around and stretching his arms, taking off his shirt, flipping it off. I have lots of memories. He was a young, young, good-looking man. If your loved one is sick, you struggle with him for years—that's different. But in just a few days, Eric was gone.

I regret so much that I didn't get to say good-bye to Eric. I think about how he told my daughter Youngor that they should wait until I came home to go to the hospital. But she was so scared that she called the ambulance. If I was there, I would have taken him to Parkland, which is the county hospital. Parkland has lots of immigrants, more than Presbyterian. Maybe he would be alive today.

Two days after Eric died, the news said that a nurse who cared for him was in quarantine. On Friday, they announced that she was in quarantine, and on Sunday, they confirmed Ebola. Then another nurse was confirmed with Ebola. People started calling me.

"See what has happened? Why are you not having it? You were his wife. You took care of the dirty clothes and yet you don't have it. What is going on?" I could not tell them. I didn't know.

Eric's nephew Josephus was so angry about his uncle's death that he wrote an editorial opinion in the *Dallas Morning News* that upset many people. He felt that Eric had been treated differently as a man of color with no insurance. He complained about the family's lack of access to Eric in the hospital. He said the hospital made many mistakes. I did not see things exactly as he did, but on some things we agreed: Eric never would knowingly expose people to Ebola, and we did not want other families to go through this experience.

These were hard words. They made people in Dallas angry and lots of letters in the newspaper showed it.

"Are you serious?"

"You have got to be kidding!"

"Someone lies to officials to come into our country with a serious illness; exposes untold people to Ebola; we hospitalize him, clean their house and then sanitize it, have to place a guard on the door so they don't wander off; and after all of these thousands of dollars, they weren't treated fairly?"

"This is a case of, 'Yeah, but what have you done for me lately?'" wrote Jan from Waxahachie.

A retired doctor wrote a letter to the newspaper saying, "To Duncan's nephew, I would ask, what level of care would he have received if he had remained in Liberia?"

"In Josephus Weeks' column he did not mention a thank-you to the people of Dallas County for picking up the tab for his uncle's costly care. Now is this a great country or what? You get free care and can complain about it, too," wrote a man named George.

"Pardon us for not being perfect people with a perfect health care system," wrote Ann, all the way from New Berlin, Wisconsin.

A letter signed by John Rice said, "The truth is, Mr. Duncan knowingly got on a plane from the hot zone of Ebola. I believe he had to at least suspect he had been in contact with the virus, but lied about it on the form."

"Why was he not taken or driven to Parkland, where they are prepared for a potential pandemic? Parkland is a county, not-for-profit, hospital."

"Call me callous, but until the race merchants like John Wiley Price and Jesse Jackson, and county judges like Clay Jenkins get out of the way and let cooler, more logical people sort this out, this stupid name calling and second-guessing will only get worse."

"Political correctness in the face of a potential epidemic is insane, but not surprising. That is the world we live in."

"To damn the good folks at Presbyterian Hospital is irresponsible, but also not surprising."

I understand why people were so angry. Many said that
the *Dallas Morning News* should not have run Josephus's letter. I was not agreeing with Josephus, but I was also angry
and hurt, wondering what I should do.

On October 16, three days after the greatest danger of
infection passed for the four of us, a man with Presbyterian
Hospital called to apologize. I didn't know his name, but he
said he spoke for the hospital.

"We did not do enough to save his life. We are deeply
sorry," he said.

"Well, Jehovah God, you have served justice," I said after
I hung up the phone.

Tomorrow belongs to God. Had it belonged to mankind,
I would not have brought Eric to America and he would not
have come here to suffer and die. He would have stayed in
his own country if he knew he was sick. But we do not know
the future. The future belongs to God. But now at least God
showed that it was not Eric's time to die. I'm glad that they
apologized.

I called Pastor George, "I am so happy. They have admitted that they were wrong. Now I can let some of it go."

"Do you want to put out a statement to the press, Louise?" Pastor George said.

And so he helped me write another one: "I am grateful
to the hospital for this personal call. I am grateful to God
that this leader reached out and took responsibility for the
hospital's actions. Hearing this information will help me as
I mourn Eric's death."

The hospital ran a big ad in the newspaper giving its
apology. Then Daniel Varga, the medical officer for Presbyterian, told Congress, "Unfortunately, in our initial

treatment of Mr. Duncan, despite our best intentions and a highly skilled medical team, we made mistakes. We did not correctly diagnose his symptoms as those of Ebola. We are deeply sorry."

Friends and family members were saying, "Sue the hospital."

But Eric's mother said, "Money cannot bring my son back." She woke me up some mornings crying. She kept saying over and over, "My son was beautiful. Now I will die, too."

Karsiah did not want to sue, either. When lawyers tried to get him to sign a paper saying he will sue, my son said he will not.

"Mama, I don't really want a lawsuit in my father's situation. I came here to go to school and learn and work for my own money. I know that people killed my father. They didn't take care of my father, but I am not going to sue for blood money.

"God knows all that happened. He will have vengeance."

Some of Eric's family members called Karsiah stupid, said they don't need him in the family. But God heard that child say what he wants. We are godly people. Eric was a godly man. We trust in God who knows everything and will punish anyone who did wrong.

# CHAPTER FOURTEEN

# *No Room at the Inn*

On October 19, 2014, at midnight, our quarantine was up. The next day we would leave the Catholic center for the first time in seventeen days. That night I was awake, fearing what would happen next. I was wondering if I could go back to work. When the quarantine first started, all I wanted was to have my old life back. But now I was very, very afraid to go back to it. Where would I go? How would people treat me?

One woman I don't even know named Carol messaged me on Facebook to call us disgusting. A man named Benjamin said that it was good that my lying, dying boyfriend was dead. A guy named Daniel on the Internet read a story that said Eric had quit his job abruptly. He wrote, "Yeah, quit his job abruptly, so he could lie and get the hell out of Dodge and come to America to get free health care and the welfare.

"He KNEW he was exposed and so did the family. They should be prosecuted and deported. Shame on you all for bringing this deadly disease to MY country. You reap what you sow, you get what you deserve. Duncan has now become 'the face of Ebola.' [T]he first person to infect my country with a LIE!" These were hurtful things to write. For the rest of my life, I will be remembering these bad things they said, but I am an American, too. Eric came here legally. We came here to work hard and have a better life.

Carol does not own America. Benjamin does not own America. Daniel does not own America.

Even people who didn't mean to be unkind were calling Eric "Patient Zero" and the face of Ebola like he wasn't a real person. At the *Washington Post,* an editorial said airports should be screening for Ebola the same way they screen for terrorists. But Eric was not a terrorist. He was a human who died from a terrible disease. He did not intend to hurt anyone, but these people were treating him like he was a disease.

In South Carolina, Todd Kincannon, a lawyer who was once a Republican Party executive director, tweeted that "people with Ebola in the U.S. need to be humanely put down immediately." Put down is what they do to animals. But some Americans weren't even treating Eric as well as they treat their animals. When someone set up a crowd-funding site to help pay Eric's hospital bills, only $50 came in during the first five days. Pets that need surgery often get thousands of crowd-funding dollars.

Pastor George had been working hard with all the media to tell the world that Eric was a human being and innocent. He was on television all over. He had three interviews with Anderson Cooper. In the first one, he said, "This is one of our members. Her name is Louise, and in this whole human drama we have to remember to try to treat people as persons before they are patients or any other kind of definition of them. We have a human tragedy here."

Why were people forgetting that we were human?

We knew that we were going to have to give the media
something as I came out of isolation. So Pastor George and
I came up with another statement:

> Tomorrow, my family and I will complete the twenty-one
> day quarantine period we were required to undergo be-
> cause of the Ebola virus in Dallas. We are so happy this is
> coming to an end, and we are so grateful that none of us
> has shown any sign of illness.
>
> Our happiness is mixed with sadness at the same time.
> My beloved fiancé, Thomas Eric Duncan, who was also the
> father of my son, Karsiah Eric Duncan, did not survive with
> us. We continue to mourn his loss and grieve the circum-
> stances that led to his death, just at the time we thought we
> were facing a happy future together.
>
> Our hearts also go out to the two brave women who
> have been infected by this terrible disease as they were
> trying to help him. We are also aware of how much this
> has affected many other people of my city, Dallas, and my
> country, the United States of America, even as it has in the
> country of my birth, Liberia. We also know that many peo-
> ple who work in Presbyterian Hospital are hurting because
> of this tragedy. We pray that God will bring healing to all in
> our community soon.
>
> We thank all people of kindness who have prayed for us
> during this time, and we join your prayers now for others
> who are suffering, too. We have lost so much, but we have
> our lives and we have our faith in God, which always gives
> us hope.
>
> Even though the quarantine is over, our time of mourn-
> ing is not over. Because of that, we ask to be given privacy
> as we seek to rebuild our home, our family, and our daily

lives. We will not give any interviews at this time. I do have a story to tell, and I look forward to telling it in my own way at the right time.

At this time, I would like to give my thanks to Mayor Mike Rawlings and Dallas County Judge Clay Jenkins for all the help and kindness they have shown me in the last three weeks. These two men have cared about me as a person. The many people who work with and for them, and also the state health workers who have cared for us, have been angels from God who have kept our spirits up through all of this. And of course I want to thank all my family, the Liberian community, and my friends at Wilshire Baptist Church. I look forward to seeing you all soon. All glory be to God.

Pastor George came early, at 9:00 a.m. on Monday, to welcome us back to the world. For the first time, he did not make the hugging signs. When Oliver opened the door, they hugged each other. Then Pastor George hugged all of us. Except for those times Timothy touched me, I had not touched anyone in twenty-one days.

We were ready to go, but not yet packed. The cleaning company had returned papers and pictures to us. Some charities had bought us soap and shampoo, some nail clippers, some clothes. We didn't have much to take.

Pastor George had talked with us about what kind of clothes we were going to need. Oliver spent much of his time in quarantine wearing long gym pants and no shirt. Jeffrey wore slippers and a sweat suit. I had some black stretch pants and a few tops. Timothy is a neat boy who always pays attention to his clothes, but his school uniforms were gone and all his other clothes. We didn't have much else. It would be cold soon. We had no sweaters, no coats.

Pastor George said, "The church will help you get new clothes and everything you need. I'll take you shopping. Where do you want to go?" Pastor George wanted everything to be good for us and said he would get us some gift cards.

"I like to go to Marshalls. That's where I find things I like," I said. But I was thinking that I could never replace things I had. Some of them I would never find again.

"I want to go to the mall," said Oliver.

"To get shoes," said Timothy. Timothy was so unhappy over all the shoes he had lost. Karsiah's winter clothes and some of his shoes had also been destroyed. Pastor George said the church would help with that, too.

On the morning we were going to leave, Judge Jenkins was there and my friend Saymendy Lloyd, who had helped me by talking to the reporters and sending me the photo of Eric in the hospital. The Catholic bishop Kevin Farrell also came that morning. He hugged us and then we held hands and prayed. Holding hands to pray is one of the nice things we had not been able to do. I thanked the bishop for taking us in when no one else in all of Dallas would.

The bishop said that when people heard we were at the Catholic center, some of them asked if we were Catholic, but he told them that our denomination was not what was most important. "We didn't help because you are Catholic," he said. "We helped because we are Catholic."

Pastor George had called John and Mig Coates from my Sunday-school class to take me to my daughter Youngor's apartment back in Vickery Meadow.

Pastor George was worried that I wouldn't be treated well in my old neighborhood. "What if they are mean to you, Louise? Are you sure you don't want to go to some other neighborhood? Maybe you should stay at the retreat center for longer," he said.

But Timothy was supposed to go back to school, and I wanted to be somewhere so that he could walk there. The Ivy Apartments would not take me back, and I had been about to move away anyway. Pastor George was talking about how we would have to rent an apartment. I didn't think any of the apartments would take us in.

Pastor George was talking to many people in Dallas about helping us: the mayor, the judge, Jewish Family Services, the Communities Foundation of Texas, and the Dallas Foundation. He was making calls and going to meetings every day. Lots of people wanted to help me, he said. Once when he was talking to a reporter, Pastor George said, "This city has been known around the world as the city that killed Kennedy. Now we have the eyes of the world on us again. Do you think we want to get this wrong?"

He and the judge asked me to itemize everything I had lost. I thought the county should pay me back for what they destroyed, but Pastor George said the county would not pay me. He said it was the same as when the Fire Department came to a house and destroyed things in putting out a fire.

"The Fire Department doesn't replace anything," he said. "Insurance does that, but you don't have insurance." Pastor George was on conference calls and in meetings about helping me every day. When the charities found out that I had a fifty-five-inch TV, they didn't want to replace it. They didn't want to replace my king-size bed.

One charity said they would help me for two months.

"Pastor George, this is not fair," I said.

He said, "We're going to take care of this through the church."

So he went back to the agency and he said, "You are treating this woman like people who haven't paid their utilities. This woman never defaulted on her rent. She never took food stamps. This is an unprecedented event. You want to make sure it's equal to everyone. I'm saying she's not the same. Our church is going to see her as an individual, and we're going to see her as a unique situation, and we're going to take care of her."

Pastor George said to me, "Everything you lost will be restored. The church will help." But others helped, too. Once they heard what Pastor George thought was fair, they said, "We will do everything we can."

When we got ready to leave the Catholic center, Oliver and Timothy went with Pastor George to the mall. Jeffrey went with Saymendy. I got in the backseat of John and Mig's Buick. I was about to leave my place of protection, and I was afraid. We couldn't see any cameras outside, but the reporters had special lenses. They took pictures through the fence, and people could see us leaving the house to get in the cars. At the gate, I could see the reporters and cameras outside. But they were off to the side and we didn't stop.

No one followed us.

It was lunchtime, so John stopped at Jakes Hamburgers. This is not too big a restaurant. I was a little afraid to go in, but not many people were there. We gave our order. I wanted just a hamburger, no fries. And Pepsi. I like Pepsi. A man was sitting at the table near us and could hear what we were saying. I could see that he was listening. In a little while he came walking by our table drinking his drink and looking at me. He didn't stop or say anything. He just looked. He knew who I was. Not many pictures had been published of me, maybe only one, from the day when we moved from the Ivy Apartments. No one could see my face well. But maybe this man heard my name; he knew who I was.

All the television stations had been talking about how we were getting out. Jakes has big televisions everywhere, which made me nervous, too. They might start talking about Eric or our family. Maybe they would show pictures of us and everyone in the whole place would start looking at me. Going for lunch was a bad idea.

Then something worse happened. John got a call from the sheriff's office. They wanted to know where we were, and they told us to stay there. A sheriff's deputy was coming. They didn't say why.

"Let's go," I told John. "We have to leave."

I had signed the paper saying that I would not leave quarantine. They had told me that I would go to jail if I left. I had done everything they'd told me. The sheriffs had been in their cars and opened the gates when we left the Catholic center. My mind told me I had done nothing wrong. But who knows what might happen?

"No," John said. "We have to wait." He was afraid to disobey the sheriffs. That made me even more scared.

I couldn't eat my hamburger. My breathing was fast and my heart was pounding. I couldn't get out. So much bad had happened, and now I didn't know what they would do.

Finally, a sheriff's deputy came in. He had on guns and a khaki uniform. He looked huge to me. Maybe John saw how scared I was because he got up and went over to the deputy and shook his hand. I watched them talking. Was the sheriff going to come over to me? He had some papers in his hand. I could hardly breathe now at all. They laughed. The deputy handed the papers to John.

John came back to our table. "He just wanted us to have your release from quarantine papers, Louise. Here they are. You're officially free."

Mig and John finished their food. I wrapped the rest of my hamburger up to take home. I was not hungry anymore.

"Before we go back to Youngor's place, let's see if we can get me into one of these apartment complexes," I told John. "We can make application and if there are any vacancies, I will have a place to go." So he pulled into one of the big ones and we parked near the manager's office. I didn't want to go in, so I asked John if he would do it.

"When you talk to them make sure you tell them who I am. Tell them Louise Troh. And let them know that I have been in quarantine," I told him. I did not want anyone to be surprised.

So John went in. He told them who I was and that I needed an apartment. They said they didn't have a vacancy but he could leave my number and they would call if something came open. We went to about three more apartments, and it was always the same. Take a number and they would call.

So John and Mig dropped me off at Youngor's apartment. She has a really good fiancé. They said we could stay there as long as we wanted. Pastor George was upset that there was no gate to keep reporters out, but I felt safer back with my family. The apartment isn't big. Two bedrooms and not big rooms. Youngor's family was six, and with the four of us, that made ten people in the apartment.

That night we were all so happy to be free and together. It was good, but still not the same as it once was. Before quarantine, friends were always coming into Youngor's house for visiting and having their hair done. But now a lot of those people did not come.

On Tuesday, Timothy and my grandchildren went back to school. Timothy was in the eighth grade, and maybe Pastor George was afraid that bigger kids would be unkind to him. He asked Max from my Sunday-school class to come to take Timothy to school and take him home. So Max showed up at our apartment on Tuesday early in the morning. But Timothy was already gone. He always walks to school, and so he walked on that day, too.

When I asked him to wait for Max, Timothy said what he always said, "I don't have Ebola. Nobody is going to bother me." And nobody did.

When he didn't come home right after school that day, I was so scared. Then I remembered that he had football practice. I worried one more day about him walking alone, but on the third day I stopped worrying. Nobody ever said anything bad to him as far as I know. His friends were glad he was back and playing on sports teams again.

In the next weeks, Pastor George and a realtor named Maria Ward were trying to get us a place to live. He went to the apartments where I had been about to move, and they said, "No. She can't come here."

He called one place after another and got turned down. Some people knew we needed a place because the media said we didn't have a home. People were calling the church saying they had houses or apartments we could have, but none of them were in Vickery Meadow. They were in Plano, which is far to the north, or Grand Prairie, which is far to the west, or Cedar Hill, which is far to the south. I don't like to drive on highways, so I would be all alone and once again afraid in such places.

"This is where I want to live," I told Pastor George, "so Timothy can walk to school."

"All right, Louise," he said. "I'll keep looking."

After about a week, he found a townhouse just a little way from my daughter's apartment. It had three bedrooms and three bathrooms and a double-car garage. It had a big living room like my other apartment, and a good kitchen for lots of cooking. Upstairs there were two bedrooms, a bathroom, and a big room for everyone to be and watch television or listen to music. I loved it.

A charity called Dwell with Dignity that makes the inside of houses nice for poor people volunteered to decorate the townhouse. They would bring everything: furniture, dishes, towels, shower curtains. One day I went to the church to meet with one of the main decorators, Lisa Robison. She had a basket of fabrics.

"We're going to make things just the way you like them," she said. "So when I put each piece of fabric in front of you, just say whether you like it, think it's just okay, or you don't like it at all."

I like deep colors: purple, red, orange.

When I would say yes to one, Lisa would say, "All right. This can be a pillow." Or "This will go nicely. Maybe for the bed."

Lisa said they would replace my pots and pans and fill the pantry with food. But I said no to that.

"I do not like canned foods. I will buy my own food."

I said no also to the pots and pans. The ones I use are big because I like to make lots of food. I would need to choose those.

At the same time when I was meeting with Lisa, my daughters and their families had come to the church to talk with Pastor George. They were all in his study down the hall on the second floor of the church. Pastor George has a nice dark study with shutters on the windows and walls covered with beautiful wood. He has bookcases filled with books against almost every wall. A big sofa, soft chairs, and a table for meetings. Little lamps light up the room; there are no lights in the ceiling. The room is not too bright, but always soft-feeling.

On the other side of the room is a tiny office with a little desk built into the wall where Pastor George writes his sermons. The desk is always clean. It is so little in there, like something a monk might like.

My daughters filed past Pastor George's assistant, Debby Burton, who sits in a little office outside his study. They wanted to find out what Pastor George intended to do. Everyone knew that he was helping me, but nobody had any details. Lawyers had been calling me to see if I wanted to sue. I didn't, but they kept calling. So I sent them to Pastor George and he talked with them. But he told my daughters that none of the lawyers were offering to do anything good for me.

People were telling me that I was giving too much power to Pastor George. But I just said, "That man was the one who came to visit me every day. He was always there for me. I trust him."

My daughters didn't want to be rude, but they also wanted to know if the church was getting money meant for me, and if Pastor George was the best person to help me. Others were saying he wasn't sharing enough information. My brother in Boston had also called Pastor George to find out what he was doing.

"We are giving Louise every bit of money that people send to us," Pastor George said. "We're also forwarding every letter."

People from all over the country, California, Washington, Ohio, even Canada had sent me letters saying they were praying for me. They said how sorry they were about Eric and how scary it was. And that they hoped good things would happen to me. Sometimes they put checks of $25 or maybe $50 in the letters. These people from all over were so kind. They showed me that the ugly people were not the only people in America. A few weeks later, I gave the church a donation to pay back to God the money those nice people had given me.

"I am paying back my vow to God," I said.

I also tried to give Pastor George some money, but he said no. "Then it wouldn't be that I did it for love, Louise," he said. And he hugged me, for real.

To my brother in Boston, he said, "I will be happy to order an accounting of everything that's been received."

But my brother said, "Oh no, Pastor. We wouldn't ask for anything like that." He was satisfied.

I did not doubt Pastor George, but a lot of talk was going around, with people asking for more information.

So they had the meeting and the girls were happier. But they still were worried that Eric was not being honored as he should be. Pastor George was hoping that Karsiah would get a settlement from Presbyterian without a lawsuit.

"Don't do things to make Presbyterian look bad," he said. "Just try to keep quiet and let's see if we can get them to do the right thing."

Everyone said, "Okay, Pastor." Maybe they were thinking that they were telling him the truth because they didn't intend to say anything. But my daughters and Oliver and some other friends were already planning to stand outside Presbyterian that night for a silent protest. My friend Saymendy organized it so that everyone was wearing red and black to recognize the pain and suffering Eric went through. These people believed they must do something for him. If no one cared enough to make some demonstration, maybe Eric's spirit would not rest.

They made signs that said, "Eric Duncan is a human," "This is where he came without his family seeing him," "Why no phone call? Why, why, why?" Presbyterian security watched them and reporters' floodlights made everything bright.

One of Youngor's friends, Janet Bright, spoke first and asked the photographers to stop showing Eric's picture on television.

A woman shouted, "How could you not save a soul if you have all the power in the world to help a person. I'm hurt! I'm hurt!"

When reporters asked Oliver what the demonstration was trying to accomplish, he said, "We're not hoping to accomplish anything. We're trying to get the message across that we're all human."

They prayed that Eric would be remembered as the good man he was, and not just someone who brought disease to America. Then they sang some godly songs and went home.

I did not go to the protest myself because I was still let-ting Pastor George speak for me. The church was going to help me with the townhouse rent until I could pay it my-self. Everything looked good. I thought I would soon have a home. Then the landlord asked for background checks on all of us. We weren't afraid because we all pay our bills. But there was some mix-up on Oliver's Social Security number. While we were trying to straighten that out, the landlord realized who we were. He didn't want to rent to us.

So Pastor George said, "Could the church buy this place from you?"

"I don't know," the man said. "It is worth a lot more than on the tax rolls because I have put so much into redoing it."

"Well, just tell us what you want for it," Pastor George said.

"I'll have to ask my wife," the landlord said. But nothing happened.

Pastor George was so stubborn. He wanted a place with three bedrooms because we have four people. We lived in a two-bedroom apartment, but Pastor George said that wasn't big enough. He wanted a place with a gate so that no one could bother me, or at least a garage that I could go into without getting out of my car if reporters were around.

He also wanted a place that was good enough and cheap enough that I could stay there. Some people said, "Just rent her something. And she can move."

Pastor George said no.

I said, "Just get me somewhere to lay my head."

But Pastor George said, "Be patient."

The county had towed my car and finally returned it. The county employees had been so rough about destroying

all our things, saying it was for safety. They said they sani-
tized my car, but a drink was still there in the car, not even
taken out and put in the trash. They had damaged the sides
and the bumper. Pastor George was so mad. The judge said
he would take care of it. But in the end, Pastor George
got someone in the church to fix it for lower cost and the
church paid.

All this time, Wilshire Baptist was getting e-mails and
letters from people who had seen Pastor George on television. They were saying, "Where can we find a church like
this one?" My own sister in Boston wanted to find such a
church. But Pastor George couldn't help her. Maybe there
aren't many churches like Wilshire.

The church got some bad e-mails from people who said
Wilshire shouldn't be helping our family. But they were
from people outside the church. Nobody in the church said
any bad thing. Nobody said anything about Eric staying in
my house before we were married. Nobody said we didn't
belong in this country. Nobody said Eric had brought Ebola
to America knowing he had it.

"Louise is one of us," Pastor George said.

I don't look like the people at Wilshire. I am black. And
most of them are white. Many of them, most of them I
think, have more education and more money. I don't even
know if anybody from Liberia except my family goes there.
But I think that God told me to join Wilshire. And maybe
the other people think so, too.

"Louise is our sister in Christ," said Pastor George. "We
love her. And we will be there for her in this terrible time."

The first Sunday that I was out of quarantine, I went to
church. It was something the reporters were all interested

in. The church was ready. The associate pastor is a man named Mark Wingfield who used to work in journalism. So he was important in dealing with reporters. They came from Italy, Canada, Mexico, and Europe—everywhere. One was from Italy, and the church found a member who spoke Italian so that newscast could have an interview in its own language. When Pastor George wasn't able to talk with all the reporters, Pastor Mark did.

They came from all the networks and many cable channels. The morning shows were all telling Pastor George that they were the best place for me to give an interview. They wanted my story because I had not talked to the media very much.

Even when I was in quarantine, the reporters and photographers were all in the church on Sunday mornings. Some visited Open Bible Sunday-school class.

One said, "Oh, I thought this would be a class for Africans."

But Pastor Mark said, "We don't have that kind of class. Louise is one of us."

On that first Sunday back in church, the lawn and parking lots were full of reporters. They came for the 8:30 service and stayed until noon. The church staff told them that cameras could come on church property, but they could not come inside. Reporters could come inside, but they should not try to talk to me.

I came to church with three of my granddaughters, Rose, who is six; Grace, who is seven; and Knowledge, who is five. These are the same girls who stayed at my apartment the first night Eric was in America. I went in the side door, but some reporters saw me, and there was video of me and the girls going into the church. I was hurrying and the girls were walking fast.

Once we were inside the door, Jay Pritchard, a Wilshire member who works with a public relations company called The Richards Group, was there to help. And so were Mark and members of the Open Bible class.

When I walked into the class, everyone yelled out, "Oh, Louise, we are so glad to see you." They were coming around hugging me and telling me how they were praying for me so much.

One woman I didn't know came up to hug me. Then she said, "I'm a reporter from the *Dallas Morning News.*"

I said, "I am not talking to reporters."

Other people heard us, and they came to tell the reporter to come outside the class and not to talk with me. She didn't come back.

Open Bible class had made a party for me with orange juice, cookies, sandwiches, brownies, cake, and all kinds of good things. Rose, Grace, and Knowledge were so happy to have some. Before the class, two people brought me a clipping from the *Dallas Morning News.* There had been so many bad letters about Eric and my family, but this was a letter that was not bad. It said:

> Louis Troh, the fiancée of the first Ebola victim in the United States, has finished her 21-day mandatory quarantine.
>
> What you don't know is that she is one of the finest, most compassionate caregivers at the senior living center where she works.
>
> She cared for my Mother who was in the Alzheimer's

unit until her death in January. She cared for her with the utmost dignity and compassion.

Louise is a hard worker and I don't believe she knowingly invited Ebola into her home.

The fact is she and her family didn't contract the disease. However, everything her family owned, except some photographs and passports has been incinerated.

She is an exceptional woman who has lost her fiancé and almost everything she had in this natural world.

I'm happy that she can return to work.

If this had happened to you or me, we would want to be treated fairly and compassionately.

I hope that our community shows compassion to Louise and her family as they return to everyday life.

Mary Overton, Preston Hollow

People in the class were asking me if I knew who this woman was, but I didn't.

"I think maybe her mother died in January," I said.

The teacher that day was the same young minister who had given the memorial service for my daughter Kebeh. In the prayer that morning, they gave thanks for me being well and back with them.

When I went to church I sat in my usual place. My nieces and my daughters were there with me. When Pastor George got up, he said, "Hello, Louise. Welcome back to Wilshire."

He was looking at me and I smiled. Then he showed them how to give the quarantine hug with his hands crossed over his chest. He said that there was only one of me and so many people are at Wilshire that maybe they should try just giving me the quarantine hug.

"If you would like to stand and turn around to that woman over there and give that woman a hug I think that would be nice," he said. And everyone did.

At the end of the service, Youngor went forward to join the church. Later, Pastor Mark told reporters that I might be the most-hugged woman in Dallas that day. They were not afraid to touch me.

That next week I was still scared to be out of my daughter's apartment much. But one day I had to go to the Wells Fargo bank. They know me at that bank, and I was nervous. But when I went in, the people who knew me were all coming out.

"Hey, Miss Louise," they were saying. "How are you? We miss you." Not one person said any bad thing to me.

Some other people were also writing to the newspaper to praise my daughter Youngor. A letter from a lady named Maude Small said, "Youngor Jallah, a nursing assistant who lives in the apartment community, is to be commended. After taking Duncan's temperature and against his will, she called 911.

"She would not let the paramedics into the apartment until they put on gloves and face masks. Later, she returned and sprayed the apartment with disinfectant. Let's keep her and her children in our prayers. It was her actions that sounded the alarm.

"Let this be a reminder that all of us should be concerned about the rest of us as long as we breathe the same air."

A registered nurse named Paula Dardaganian wrote, "Believing I had read every word in print and heard most TV news about the Ebola story, it wasn't until I read Maude

Small's letter that I became aware of Youngor Jallah, the nursing assistant who used the best of her knowledge to help Mr. Duncan.

"She followed good medical procedure before, when and after she called 911. She was especially astute beginning the initial care, providing information to paramedics and following up that day.

"It is good to know of Youngor Jallah's knowledgeable and courageous actions."

Others were writing to say how sad they were for our loss. For every terrible letter, there was a good one.

When the week started, I thought it was going to be good. But then disappointment. After I was rejected for the townhouse I loved, the realtor found a house to rent. I always dream of living in a house.

So I said, "Yes. This would be good."

But when the landlady realized who we were, she said, "No. I don't want to rent to them."

"They have been cleared by the county. They are completely well and there's no possibility that they have anything," Pastor George said.

"That may be," the woman said, "but they will have other Liberians coming to visit. And one of them might have Ebola. If that happened, I'd never be able to rent my house again. I'd lose my investment."

So Pastor George began to ask people at Wilshire if they could help. He started to call his friends. One of them owned a house near where I wanted to live.

It was a lovely house with brick and a yard that had hedges around it. There were three bedrooms. A garage. My grandchildren could play in the yard. But the landlord decided he needed to sell the place, not rent it. He didn't want to sell to us.

I was feeling so bad. Everyone was rejecting us. It was so crowded at Youngor's. It was getting cold, and I didn't even have a coat. People in the Liberian community wanted to help. They said that Pastor George needed to open it up so that they could find me a place.

He was trying to do it all. Reporters were calling, saying that they would help me if I would just give interviews. So I called Pastor George to tell him that this was taking too long. I needed to let other people know so they could help me. But he would not change his mind.

"If you go to the media and start complaining," he said, "two things are going to happen. The first thing is you may get a lot of people that want to help you, but you have already told me that you want to live in the Vickery Meadow community. If they call and have places to rent to you and you tell them no, then the word's going to get out that many people were willing to help, but you would not accept.

"The second thing, it will make it harder for the groups who want to help you financially. We want them to know that they are making this happen. If they think everyone else is helping, they will think you don't need it."

Oh, but I was getting impatient with Pastor George. He was impatient with me too, sometimes.

"I am working every day for you, Louise," he said. "I have another job but working for you is taking every day."

At Halloween he went to San Antonio with his wife, Kim, to see their grandchildren. Kim had to drive so that he could be on the phone all the time texting and talking about me. Media were still calling. Lawyers. And all the time, he was trying to get me a place.

"It doesn't matter how long it takes us, we're going to get this done. We will find you a good place to live," Pastor George said. Men of God can be stubborn.

Pastor George was also hearing from people who thought he was going to be sorry he had stuck with us so long. When Jesse Jackson came to Dallas and started talking about racism, he didn't come to see me or Pastor George. But talking about race gets people nervous. Some friends of Pastor George were saying to him that he was going to be the big white target if black people started to think he was protecting Presbyterian instead of me.

Those people said, "Get her a lawyer and back away."

Other people were coming from another direction, saying that I was getting too much help. I was a poor woman, a refugee. How much could I have lost? they said. I didn't have much in the first place. Why should I have a better place to live than before?

Pastor George was tired. And people were telling him he was wrong. But he said, "This is what advocacy is."

It had been almost three weeks since we left quarantine. County Judge Jenkins won reelection but he didn't get as many votes as everyone expected.

"A lot of people were mad still," he said.

I knew he meant at least partly about how he treated us so good. Eric's family in North Carolina had hired a lawyer even without Karsiah's signature. Presbyterian Hospital made a settlement that gave money to Eric's mother, father, and his four children, a twenty-two-year-old daughter in Liberia, a twelve-year-old daughter in Ghana, an eighteen-year-old son in North Carolina, and Karsiah.

The hospital also set up a foundation in Eric's name. Eric's nephew Josephus started saying good things about

Presbyterian Hospital. "If I got sick and Presbyterian was close to me, I would go there and get treated for it," he said.

Texas limits damages in these cases to $250,000. The amount each person got in the settlement is secret. But Presbyterian was more generous than the law requires.

The lawyer told reporters that I was not in the settlement because I was just Eric's fiancée and not his wife. Only wives have rights under Texas law. I did not make any public statement about that.

My son and I brought Eric to America without any help from his family. They denied that I was a wife, saying I was only a girlfriend. I'm glad that this girlfriend could be so faithful to Eric. I was not part of the settlement. That was the small deal. But I was part of the big deal, our son. I still have that part of Eric that is Karsiah. Our son is the big deal.

Meanwhile, I was still homeless. The ten people living at Youngor's were ready to have more room. I was starting to grumble.

Then my son in Liberia called me. He said, "I've been reading the Bible. I don't know a lot but I am thinking that one thing is for sure in the Bible. Do not curse the prophet of God. Respect the prophet of God. It would be a very bad thing, displeasing to God for anyone to curse the prophet of God."

I knew that my son was speaking the truth. So when anyone called me to say that I should not respect Pastor George, I told them I would keep trusting him.

Pastor George's friend at Wilshire who had decided not to rent or sell his house to us did not forget that we needed help. He found a two-story condo in Vickery Meadow. The owner wanted $75,000. So Pastor George asked that man and two other Wilshire members to put up $25,000. My friend Max from the Open Bible class was one of them. I would rent the condo from these men. The church would pay some rent, and then when I could go back to work, I would start paying. But first the homeowner's association had to approve us.

Pastor George was so unhappy with this idea of getting approval. "They all say no if we tell them," he told the investors. "Everybody I run into tells me yes and then they tell me no. Are they going to say no, too?"

But the investors said they wanted the approval of the board. And they must tell the board who we were. So a meeting was held, and something unusual happened.

When the representative of the board heard that it was Louise Troh, the fiancée of Eric Duncan, and her boys, he said, "This is something that we want to do. I will work to make sure there is approval."

And so they said okay. The condo wasn't perfect. The courtyard had rocks and dirt in it. The walls were dirty inside. Some wires were sticking out of the wall. But another man from Wilshire sent in crews to clean the windows and paint, fix the walls, and clean up.

The next week, in came the Dwell with Dignity women with sewing machines, hammers, screwdrivers, towels and linens, and supplies and furniture. For four days they worked. And no one was allowed to see what they were doing.

# CHAPTER FIFTEEN

# Chasing Away Darkness

At last my new condo was ready. Pastor George kept saying, "Don't come up until the place is decorated. It's going to look so pretty."

We were to gather at 4:00 p.m. on a Thursday. The Dwell with Dignity ladies had kept it all so secret. They wanted everyone to see at once what they'd done. Judge Jenkins was there and so was Stanley Gaye from the Liberian Community Association of Dallas/Fort Worth. And of course Pastor George was there.

Fresh flowers were in the dining room and potted plants were in the courtyards. My room had a king-size bed so my grandchildren could sleep with me. The ladies had made pillows, curtains, and bedding from the fabrics I picked. They had installed a fifty-five-inch television in the living room. Timothy had his own room with a big "T" over the bed. Oliver and Jeffrey had twin beds with trundle beds underneath so other people could sleep over. In the bathrooms were towels, shower curtains, and nice rugs. In the kitchen were dishes and silverware and glasses. I had never lived in such a lovely place. And it was just exactly how Pastor George said it would be.

When my family and I came through the door, my daughters were singing, "My Jesus he never fails. I said my Jesus he never fails. I said my Jesus he never fails."

When I saw all the beautiful things, I was crying for joy. Pastor George had us all join hands while he thanked God for all He'd given us. I thanked everyone in the room. One by one.

Then I said, "I thank you all from my heart. I pray that for the great kindness you have shown my family each and every one of you will be blessed by God now and to the fourth generation."

Everybody had helped me in this time of crisis. I am so happy that God gave me a second chance and that these really good people treated me like a human being.

Pastor George was right about being patient and not saying things that had not been proven. Even though many people believe bad things about Presbyterian, I did not say anything to the public. Pastor George and I worked with a malpractice lawyer, Stephen Malouf, who volunteered to help us. He said that we could try to establish that I was Eric's wife under Liberian community law and entitled to damages. But it would be a long, hard trial. I decided I did not want to sue.

Two days later, on November 16, we held Eric's memorial service. Two memorial services had been held for Eric, the one in North Carolina before I came out of quarantine, and the one at Wilshire on his death day, also when I was in quarantine. But I had not been able to attend them. I needed to attend a service myself. My heart was still so aching for Eric. I didn't know how to go on. I couldn't think about what to do next.

And so Pastor George said, "Of course, Louise. We must have a memorial service at Wilshire."

The minister who does the music was there to sing, and so was my Liberian friend who has the same name as my Liberian daughter who died, Kebeh. She sang a hymn. Oliver Smallwood, Eric's nephew, who had been so afraid of being sick with Ebola, read a statement from Eric's mother.

"My child was so beautiful," Oliver read. "I will miss him forever."

Bishop Nathan Kortu prayed to Almighty God. We all lifted our hands to heaven. I shut my eyes and cried. The bishop said, "The devil lost, Almighty God beat him back. Through Eric Duncan the devil was defeated. Eric helped a pregnant girl and because of that he contracted Ebola. People had been dying of Ebola but the world did not know it. Then Eric Duncan came to America. When he became sick with Ebola, the world paid attention. Now the world is helping Liberia fight Ebola. The devil lost. Praise God."

The Bishop's words were so true. The support in fighting against Ebola was so important that I believe Africa ought to honor the day Eric's death was announced by having a moment of silence across the continent every year.

Pastor George spoke.

"After being a mere human being among the 7 billion on the planet, Eric became the face of Ebola, the symbol of a disease that takes the life of nearly half of those who contract it. When you are a symbol of something, you become subject to what other people want to say you mean. We have tried to remind people all along that Eric Duncan was a man first and foremost, and that there are limits of decency to what anyone will make of another person's life who cannot speak for himself."

"Eric Duncan had Ebola. Eric Duncan was not Ebola. Person more than patient. Man more than disease."

I nodded; so much I wanted people to remember this. Eric was a kind man, a gentle man who never would have infected me or anyone in my family with a deadly disease. People forget: he sat in the front seat of that taxi that took the pregnant girl to the hospital. No one thought she had the virus, only that she died in childbirth, same as my daughter Kebeh.

"Over and over, Louise has used spiritual language to talk about her sadness and grief. We said in the quarantine house that how we all acted in response to this would be a witness. When she spoke of forgiveness and mercy, compassion and kindness, leaving vengeance to God and judgment to heaven, she did so because she saw Eric's death and her suffering from inside the story of Christ. The light of Christ shone from within, chasing away the darkness."

*Yes, yes, Pastor George, that is how it was,* I thought. *The words of the Bible are the truth.*

"It was the power of God within earthen vessels, as Paul put it. Afflicted but not crushed. Perplexed but not despairing. Persecuted but not forsaken. Struck down but not destroyed. Always carrying around the awareness of the death of Christ, so that we might feel the power of his resurrection, too."

"So we do not lose hope. Eric did not suffer alone; he suffered inside the suffering of his Savior. Louise did not suffer alone, she suffered inside the suffering of her Savior. And because of that, they could go on—Eric to be with the

Lord and let go to this life too soon. Louise to be with the Lord still in this life, knowing that suffering is for a time, love and life and joy for eternity."

After the service, my friends came up to greet me. And to them I said, "I'm back. Eric was the sacrifice. I was the witness for what it is to be Christian." I was rejoining life.

I was at peace. At last.

It is the custom among Liberians to have a T-shirt made to honor the loved one who has passed. The T-shirt has photos of the person and some writing. Mourners buy those shirts and wear them to honor the dead. The T-shirts for my Liberian daughter Kebeh have been lost forever, burned with all my other possessions. But Jeffrey had worked on his computer for weeks so we would have a T-shirt for Eric.

It has a picture of him in the Ivory Coast when he was so young. He was wearing shades and looking so cool. Then Jeffrey took the photo of Eric that the reporters got from Facebook, the one with the bright green shirt that everyone in the world had seen. The rest of the world will never know Eric in any other clothes, but we did not want that look to be the one on his T-shirt. Jeffrey changed the shirt for a black suit coat, white shirt, and a red and blue tie so that Eric now looked dignified and even more handsome.

We thought for a long time about what words to put on the T-shirt. On the front we put, "It's difficult to accept death in this society because it is so unfamiliar. In spite of the fact that it happens all the time, we never see it . . ."

Yes, Eric was the face of Ebola. He helped the world see the death of thousands of Africans. Over 7,500 have died. On the back of the T-shirt are these words: "Some memory never ends, my love for you never dies. And my tears for you will never be dried."

I had many fears and many questions about what happened at Presbyterian Hospital, but I am putting those things away. God alone knows what really happened. Underneath Eric's picture I put the words that Pastor George and I said so many times during my dark days.

"Vengeance belongs to God."

And then, "May your soul rest in peace."

## ACKNOWLEDGMENTS

I would like to thank God first, then my Christian brothers and sisters and all God's faithful children. I thank Presbyterian Hospital, Dallas County, and the state of Texas, and all my relatives, friends, and loved ones, including my grandkids and my children. I especially thank my son Timothy, who went through all this with me. I would like to thank all my fellow Africans and all the people who prayed for me. I am very grateful to the Garland Church of Pentecost that raised money to help me and the brother, Rex, who brought the money. I want to thank the Open Bible class at Wilshire Baptist Church, and all the people at Wilshire. I thank Pastor George and Pastor Mark, who did so much for me. The whole church was so good to me, including those little children who wrote me some encouraging letters, praying for blessings for me each day, telling me they were all with me in spirit.

I appreciate Judge Jenkins and Mayor Rawlings and all the health workers who were not afraid to come to help me, especially Sonya Hughes, who was so good to me. I thank the Catholic Diocese of Dallas for giving me a home and the Liberian Community Association of Dallas/Fort Worth, the president and all the members. I am also more grateful than I can say to Scott Mendel, Amanda Murray, Patricia Mulcahy, Georgina Levitt, and Kathleen Schmidt for their wonderful professionalism and great work on this project. Thank you also to Christine Marra at *Marra*thon, whose unfailing diligence and good cheer made hard work so much easier. I would especially like to thank Harvey Weinstein for believing in my story. And last, I'd like to thank Christine Wicker, without whom this book might never have been written.

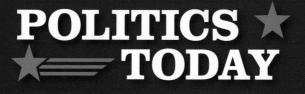

# POLITICS TODAY

# WHO ARE 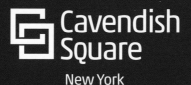 PROGRESSIVES

## and What Do They Believe In?

Matt Bougie

Cavendish Square

New York

Published in 2020 by Cavendish Square Publishing, LLC
243 5th Avenue, Suite 136, New York, NY 10016

Copyright © 2020 by Cavendish Square Publishing, LLC
First Edition

No part of this publication may be reproduced, stored in a retrieval system, or transmitted in any
form or by any means—electronic, mechanical, photocopying, recording, or otherwise—without the
prior permission of the copyright owner. Request for permission should be addressed to Permissions,
Cavendish Square Publishing, 243 5th Avenue, Suite 136, New York, NY 10016. Tel (877) 980-4450; fax
(877) 980-4454.

Website: cavendishsq.com

This publication represents the opinions and views of the author based on his or her personal
experience, knowledge, and research. The information in this book serves as a general guide only. The
author and publisher have used their best efforts in preparing this book and disclaim liability rising
directly or indirectly from the use and application of this book.

All websites were available and accurate when this book was sent to press.

Library of Congress Cataloging-in-Publication Data

Names: Bougie, Matt, author.
Title: Who are progressives and what do they believe in? / Matt Bougie.
Description: New York : Cavendish Square, [2019] | Series: Politics today |
Audience: Grades 7-12. | Includes bibliographical references and index.
Identifiers: LCCN 2018057025 (print) | LCCN 2019000317 (ebook) | ISBN 9781502645234 (ebook) |
ISBN 9781502645227 (library bound) | ISBN 9781502645210 (pbk.)
Subjects: LCSH: Democratic Party (U.S.) | Progressivism (United States politics)--Juvenile literature. |
United States--Politics and government--Juvenile literature.
Classification: LCC JK2316 (ebook) | LCC JK2316 .B69 2019 (print) | DDC 320.51/30973--dc23
LC record available at https://lccn.loc.gov/2018057025

Editorial Director: David McNamara
Editor: Erin L. McCoy
Copy Editor: Nathan Heidelberger
Associate Art Director: Alan Sliwinski
Designer: Jessica Nevins
Production Coordinator: Karol Szymczuk
Photo Research: J8 Media

The photographs in this book are used by permission and through the courtesy of: Cover (left
column- top to bottom) AXL/Shutterstock.com, Lane V. Erickson/Shutterstock.com, 3dfoto/
Shutterstock.com, (right) Tatsuya Ohinata/Shutterstock.com; p. 4 GraphicaArtis/Getty Images; p.
7 American Press Association, Library of Congress/File: Rockefellers.png/Wikimedia Commons/
Public Domain; p. 8 The Yorck Project (2002) 10.000 Meisterwerke der Malerei (DVD-ROM),
distributed by DIRECTMEDIA Publishing GmbH. ISBN: 3936122202/File: Allan Ramsay 003.jpg/
Wikimedia Commons/Public Domain; p. 9. L'Histoire par l'image (http://www.histoire image.org/
site/oeuvre/analyse.php?i=140&d=1&v=1789&w=1789)/File: Anonymous, Prise de la Bastille.jpg/
Wikimedia Commons/Public Domain; p. 11 Scanned by the Seattle Public Library/File: Can factory
workers stamping out end discs, published 1909.jpg/Wikimedia Commons/Public Domain; p. 16
Senate TV/AP Images; p. 18 Michael Vadon, own work/File: Senator of Vermont Bernie Sanders at
Derry Town Hall, Pinkerton Academy NH October 30th, 2015, 06.jpg/Wikimedia Commons/CCA-
SA 4.0 International; p. 21 Underwood & Underwood, Library of Congress/File: Muir and Roosevelt
restored.jpg/Public Domain; p. 22 National Photo Company Collection, Library of Congress/File:
Robert LaFollette LCCN2002695701.jpg/Wikimedia Commons/Public Domain; p. 23 Spartan7W,
own work/File: Progressive Moose walking.png/Wikimedia Commons/CCA-SA 4.0 International;
p. 25 Paul Schutzer/The LIFE Picture Collection/Getty Images; p. 28 Cate Gillon/Getty Images; p.
30 Author unknown/U.S. National Archives and Records Administration/File: Depression, Breadlines,
New York City, NARA 196499.tif/Wikimedia Commons/Public Domain; p. 33 Bettmann/Getty
Images; p. 34 Author unknown, Library of Congress/File: Upton Sinclair cph.3c32336.jpg/Wikimedia
Commons/Public Domain; p. 36 Ullstein Bild/Getty Images; p. 39 Everett Historical/Shutterstock.com;
p. 41 Amy Osborne/AFP/Getty Images; p. 42 Tom Williams/CQ Roll Call/Getty Images; p. 44 David
Hume Kennerly/Getty Images; p. 46 Don Emmert/AFP/Getty Images; p. 47 Nic Neufeld/Shutterstock.
com; p. 48 Transferred to Commons by Maksim/map by Brion Vibbers/File: Nordic-countries.png/
Wikimedia Commons/CCA-SA 3.0 Unported.

Printed in the United States of America

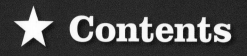

# Contents

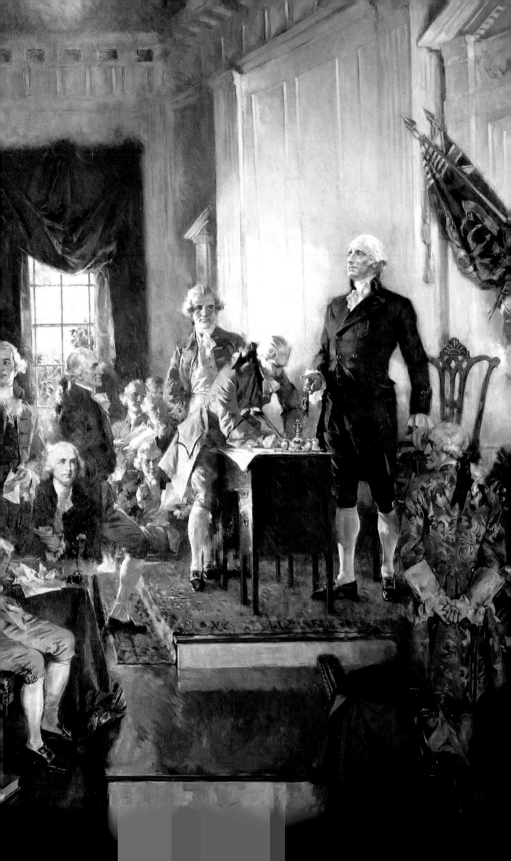

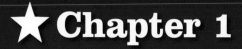

# ★ Chapter 1

# What Makes a Progressive

The progressive ideology has a long history in the United States and around the world, dating back to its earliest appearances during the Enlightenment and the Industrial Revolution. Progressivism remains an influential political movement to this day. To understand this ideology, we must learn how it has manifested during its long history—and begin with a clear understanding of what an ideology is.

## Defining the Progressive Ideology

An ideology is an overarching system of thought and belief that shapes political and moral philosophy. When someone has an ideology, they tend to think that society and government should operate in a way that reflects this ideology. Because of this belief, they tend to support policies and laws that encourage people to act in a way that fits within their chosen ideology.

Ideologies often arise in opposition to something. Great thinkers, philosophers, economists, or everyday people see a problem with their world and try to think of how the

*Opposite*: George Washington presides over the signing of the US Constitution in Philadelphia in 1787.

world ought to be or how they could solve this fundamental problem that they see. They form theories and look for examples to prove that their ideas are worthwhile, and then they try to influence others to see how an ideological shift could improve the world. There are many different ideologies that claim that they can solve many of the world's problems.

Progressivism is an ideology that, generally speaking, supports change and moving forward. While people who identify as progressives come from many different backgrounds and are demographically diverse, there are a few things that they all share.

First, progressives in the United States believe that the government should change and evolve based on what is occurring in the world. They believe that the US Constitution, a document written in the late eighteenth century, can and should be interpreted in a way that reflects modern society. People who view the Constitution this way are called instrumentalists. On the other side are formalists, who believe that the Constitution should only be interpreted in the way that its original writers intended.

Second, progressives have traditionally believed that capitalism and the pursuit of wealth inevitably do more harm than good to the vast majority of people. Progressives should not be considered revolutionaries, however, because they do not want to see capitalism completely overturned. Instead, they want to alleviate some of the worst versions of excess and exploitation that capitalism fosters, and replace the strong individualism of current capitalistic society with a system that is more cooperative and democratic. Beyond working toward economic reforms, progressives also want to reform cultural norms, bringing a greater sense of justice and fairness to society.

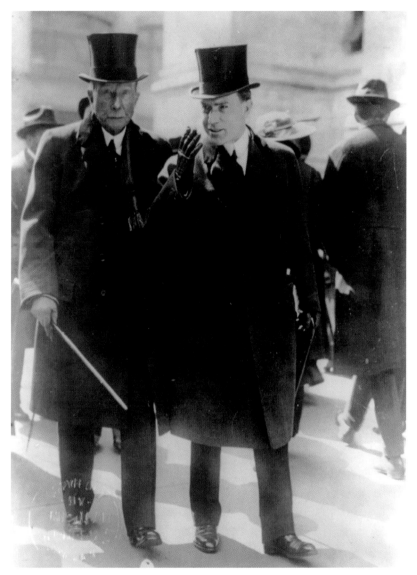

John D. Rockefeller (*left*), pictured with his son, was a wealthy American industrialist.

Specific policies and courses of action arise from these beliefs, and these policies attempt to achieve overarching goals. Progressives want a strong federal government that has the ability to make laws that protect the environment, create business regulations that favor the laboring class, and take a higher rate of taxes from people who earn more money. They also push legislators to protect the civil rights of marginalized groups and prevent discrimination against these people.

## Where Does Progressivism Come From?

Like many aspects of American culture and government, progressivism has its foundation in European philosophy, specifically in Enlightenment-era philosophers. The Enlightenment was a movement that started in Europe in the late 1600s and continued throughout the 1700s. It rejected the strict, dogmatic principles of religion and instead focused on emerging scientific theories that offered a different, empirical explanation of natural phenomena. Instead of accepting explanations that couldn't be proven or disproven, certain philosophers turned to science as a way to explain how the natural world worked.

It wasn't long before political philosophers began applying this rationalist philosophy to society. Much in the way that the Catholic Church maintained power by appealing to a heavenly decree,

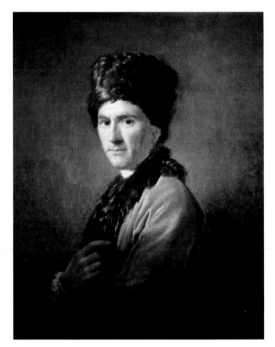

Jean-Jacques Rousseau was an Enlightenment-era philosopher whose ideas influenced progressivism.

kings and queens of that time were seen as being put in place by God. Thinkers such as Voltaire and Jean-Jacques Rousseau began pushing for a society that was not dictated by Catholicism and wasn't controlled by a divinely appointed monarch. Instead, they advocated a system that was more dictated by the people.

Civil unrest began to grow, and revolutions that undermined the wealthy ruling class started springing up in France, England, and the American colonies. Violent revolutions overthrew monarchies and gave rise to representative democracies. People who were once alienated from the political process were suddenly able to vote for policies and representatives who they believed would fight on their behalf. Once the working class was finally part of the political process, they began to divide into groups to pursue

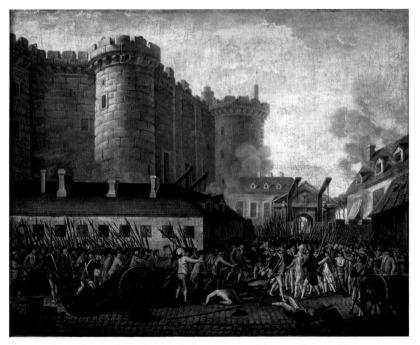

The French Revolution, shown here with the storming of the Bastille in 1789, was a working-class uprising against the French upper class.

the policies that they felt would be most advantageous. While some preferred a system close to the monarchy, others wanted to keep pushing for more political power so they could continue an agenda that favored the working class.

## Progressivism in the United States

Progressivism in the United States began to flourish as a response to modernization and the ways the Industrial Revolution was changing American capitalism. Factories allowed a lot of goods to be produced cheaply and quickly, but there were consequences to this new speed. Labor became unspecialized because a person no longer needed to know how to create a product from start to finish. Instead of a craftsperson taking a long time to create every single piece of a barrel or a cart, a factory could break the process down into many small tasks and get each worker to perform one of the smaller tasks very quickly, over and over again. This caused people to become disconnected from the work that they did, and it allowed those who owned the factories to make a lot of money.

This mass production led to waste and widespread consumption of natural resources. Meanwhile, workers toiled in unsafe conditions for little money, and there was suddenly a class of incredibly wealthy people who owned the factories and ran the large corporations. Some people who saw this disparity in wealth believed that there could be a better way, in which people who worked in the factories would have more of a say and a larger share of the profits. These people were called progressives. Progressives believed that this vast wealth was built on the backs of the lower and middle class, and that this system was designed to keep workers subservient to the wealthy. Seeing this system as a detriment

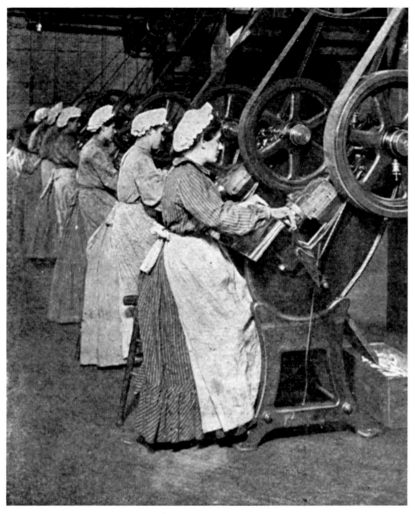

Women work in an H. J. Heinz can factory, circa 1909. Women as well as men worked long hours in factories for low wages during this era of US history.

to the interests of the majority of the population, they began to organize to change laws.

Around these common interests, writers and politicians came together to create the Progressive Party, focused on strengthening workers' rights and preserving natural resources for the enjoyment of all people. The party enjoyed

Because progressivism is not itself a political party, it's difficult to get specific demographic information about who considers themselves progressive. Political parties are formed around a belief in specific policies and approaches to government. As a party's fundamental ideologies shift, we often see members leave the party and become independent voters, or even defect to the other major political party out of anger or frustration. In American politics today, conservatism is generally associated with the Republican Party, and liberalism is associated with the Democratic Party. But although many use the terms "liberal" and "progressive" interchangeably, not all Democrats can be considered progressives.

Progressives today often support such policies as marijuana legalization, prison reform, and legalization of gay marriage. Economically, liberals and progressives alike tend to favor higher corporate taxes and a stronger social safety net for lower-income individuals. In 2016, identifying as progressive also meant supporting health-care reform and promoting government regulation of the health-care industry. Democrats who see themselves as moderate or conservative rather than liberal are likely to identify as such because they oppose these more progressive policies.

Whites make up the majority of Americans, and they also make up the majority of Democratic voters. However, 63 percent of Hispanic voters, 84 percent of African American voters, and 65 percent of Asian American voters identify as Democrats. Slightly more women than men identify as Democrats across all racial groups.

In 2016, Gallup researchers polled registered Democrats on whether or not they identified as "liberal" as opposed to "moderate" or "conservative." The poll found that 44 percent of all Democrats identified as "liberal," which was a significant shift toward liberalism compared to previous polls. In 2001, only 30 percent of all Democrats identified as liberal. This shift signals that progressive ideas are likely becoming more important to the future of the Democratic Party.

The most significant movement toward the liberal ideology was among non-Hispanic whites and older Democrats. The number of white Democrats who identified as liberal increased sharply from 2001 to 2016. In 2016, 50 percent of white Democrats considered themselves to be liberal, while only 36 percent of nonwhite and Hispanic Democrats considered themselves liberal.

Education level, geography, and age are also correlated with ideology. Democrats with a higher level of education are more likely to self-identify as liberal, while less-educated Democrats resist the label. Democrats who live in the Western states are most likely to be progressive, while Southern Democrats are less likely to be progressive. Younger voters are much more likely to support progressive policies than older Democrats, but there has also been a significant shift leftward among older Democratic voters.

These shifting demographics show that progressive ideologies are taking a more prominent role in how the Democratic Party selects candidates and the types of policies they are looking to pursue. While previous iterations of the Democratic Party might have been more willing to compromise on such issues as corporate tax cuts and the loosening of environmental regulations, the new, more progressive party may not be so willing to negotiate.

some minor successes in local and state governments before rising to national prominence when it selected former president Theodore Roosevelt to be its candidate in the 1912 presidential election. The Progressive Party effectively split the Republican Party, drawing away many former Republican voters and allowing Democrat Woodrow Wilson to claim the presidency. After this, the Progressive Party fell out of favor as the more pressing concerns of World War I took over.

In modern times, progressive policies have been implemented by liberal-leaning legislatures and presidents. The modern progressive movement was thrust back into the public consciousness by the 2007–2009 financial crisis. As the financial industry pursued record profits in the early twenty-first century, firms began making risky financial investments without taking the appropriate precautions. While most of this was legal, it ended up being very costly for the country. In the wake of the financial collapse, many middle-class families felt the negative effects of the market crash. Because the crisis affected so many people, the government began passing laws to reform the financial industry and try to prevent this type of crisis from happening again. In 2010, President Barack Obama signed the Dodd-Frank Act. The law's intention was to "promote the financial stability of the United States by improving accountability and transparency in the financial system." In its efforts to implement checks and balances on powerful institutions, it could be considered a progressive piece of legislation.

Further progressive reforms took place in 2010 with the passing of the Affordable Care Act, which made health-care coverage more accessible to millions of Americans. Likewise, pushes to increase the minimum wage could be considered progressive. Many of these reforms have met with resistance from conservatives, who tend to support traditional ideals and oppose government intervention into everyday life.

In the aftermath of the 2016 presidential election, many of these reforms are being targeted for repeal or replacement by the Donald Trump administration and by the US Congress, which was Republican-controlled for the first two years of Trump's presidency. For example, there have been numerous attempts to repeal the Affordable Care Act, and the Dodd-Frank Act has been targeted for repeal by President Trump. Conservatives see these reforms as overreaching and unhelpful to businesses, and they believe that the markets can and should regulate themselves.

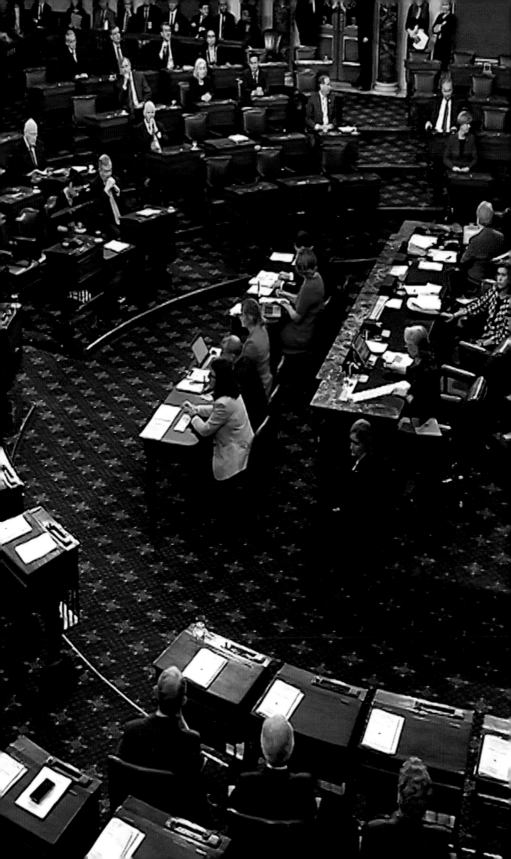

# ★ Chapter 2

# Progressivism, Politics, and Government

From the earliest days of progressivism, supporters of this ideology have sought to change the fundamental structures of government. They have usually pursued legislation that empowers and supports the working class while preventing too much wealth from being concentrated in the hands of a few powerful people. This has generally met with resistance from conservatives, moderates, and some liberals, who argue that progressivism moves too far away from capitalist ideals, or supports social change that is at odds with traditional American values.

## Progressives and the Party System

In a republic such as the United States, populations elect representatives to promote their interests at all levels of government. When someone wants to become one of these representatives, he or she campaigns and meets voters while having conversations and determining what the voters want most from their government. These representatives can operate at the local, state, and federal level, and in each of

*Opposite*: The Senate Chamber is shown in this Senate TV video still from October 5, 2018, during a procedural vote on the nomination of Brett Kavanaugh to the US Supreme Court.

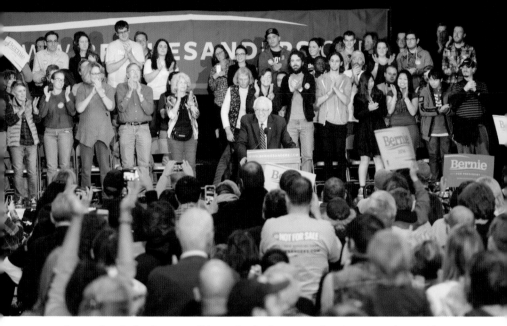

Senator Bernie Sanders, a candidate to be the Democratic Party's nominee for president, speaks at a town hall meeting in New Hampshire on October 30, 2015.

these levels they have different responsibilities, as well as different agendas that they pursue.

As representatives work to achieve the goals that their constituents elected them to pursue, they collaborate with other representatives who share similar goals. Likewise, if representatives believe that a certain behavior is immoral or wrong, they can work together to get laws passed to make it illegal.

Representatives who work together to achieve common goals are often part of the same political party. The most prominent political parties in the United States are the Republican Party and the Democratic Party. Republicans generally represent the more conservative citizens and Democrats the more liberal citizens. Conservatives tend to believe that the government should be small, should have limited power within the economy, and shouldn't pursue legislation related to a citizen's private life. Liberals tend to believe in more government intervention—for instance, in regulating what corporations can and cannot do—while passing laws that grant greater protections to lower- and middle-class citizens, especially to groups who are, or who in the past have been, oppressed or discriminated against.

Within each of these parties there are people who hold different ideologies; some people, meanwhile, hold beliefs that don't fit within either of these parties. For example, some people identify as libertarian—believing that the government should be incredibly limited in economic matters and in shaping national policies. Libertarians tend to align themselves with the Republican Party because Republicans generally favor the same small-government approach that libertarians do. However, not all Republicans are libertarian, and not all libertarians are Republicans.

Likewise, progressives tend to align themselves with the Democratic Party because of their shared belief in a strong federal government that guarantees social and political rights to all groups. Progressives and Democrats also agree that taxes are an effective means to fund public projects. But again, not all progressives are Democrats, and not all Democrats are progressives.

Progressives in the United States tend to favor social programs that fight back against inequality and injustice. Sometimes, they pursue laws that other, more conservative people may deem immoral, unnecessary, or wrong. In the past, progressives have pushed for women's suffrage, prisoners' rights, and civil rights for African Americans and other marginalized groups with the goal of ensuring equitable treatment for all people. Progressives have also taken up causes related to gender equality, legalized abortion, minimum wage increases, and affirmative action. These causes align with the progressive idea that all people should have the same level of opportunity and liberty.

Some liberals may not favor as much government regulation of business as progressives do but still support progressive social reforms. These people would not be considered progressives because a key part of the progressive platform is economic reform. In the same sense, liberals who believe that the government should impose heavy taxes on corporations but do not support progressive social legislation would not be considered progressive because social reform is an important part of the ideology.

## The Progressive Party in the Early 1900s

A political party is usually comprised of a variety of factions: groups of people with differing ideologies or ideas of how that party should operate. Sometimes, these factions differ enough on key points to cause an ideological split within the party. The Progressive Party arose from one such schism within the Republican Party in the early 1900s.

During Abraham Lincoln's presidency, the Republican Party became the party of social reform by passing legislation to end slavery and prevent further exploitation of African Americans. However, as the Republican Party grew and attracted more and more people, competing ideologies emerged. While most Republicans supported such reforms, some wanted to scale them back or were willing to compromise on some of them in a bid to keep political power. Theodore Roosevelt was at the center of this ideological split.

Roosevelt became president after William McKinley was assassinated in September 1901. During the latter part of his second term, Roosevelt began to pursue policies that were considered quite progressive, especially for the time. For instance, he established the US Forest Service and designated several large swaths of land to be reserved as national parks, where businesses could not move in and extract natural resources. These parks would be maintained and preserved for the enjoyment of all citizens.

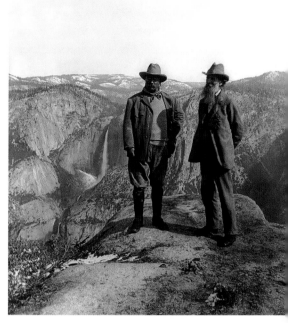

Theodore Roosevelt (*left*) is pictured with renowned naturalist John Muir in Yosemite National Park in 1906.

Roosevelt also signed significant consumer-protection laws. In 1906, the public became very worried about what types of foreign substances were in the packaged foods they were consuming. Journalistic reports of the hazardous and disgusting materials that contaminated many factory-made foods caused an outcry, and Roosevelt signed the Pure Food and Drug Act of 1906 to prevent mislabeled food and to establish government inspections of food to ensure quality. These progressive reforms changed the way that businesses operated and allowed for greater government oversight of these industries. The law also paved the way for further reforms.

Theodore Roosevelt honored his promise to step down after completing his second term as president, and

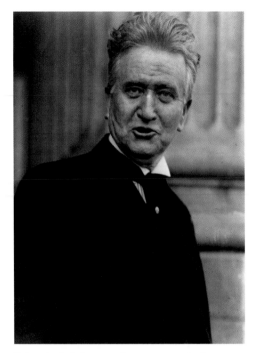

Robert La Follette was a fierce opponent of corporations and fought government corruption.

Republican William Howard Taft was elected president in 1908. After ascending to power, however, Taft and the Republican Party became more conservative and did not push the progressive agenda that Roosevelt and earlier Republicans had pursued. Roosevelt believed strongly in the preservation of natural resources and supported legislation to control the power of corporations and to protect consumers from bad business practices. When Taft's presidency failed to pursue these agendas, Roosevelt looked elsewhere to enact change. He began campaigning with the Progressive Party, a group that had splintered from the Republican Party in the late 1800s when Robert "Fighting Bob" La Follette declared that the Republican Party was no longer serving the interests of the people it represented. Roosevelt drew excitement around and attention to a political party that had not gotten much traction nationally.

La Follette was a politician from Wisconsin who held many different offices during his life. He served as a member of Congress in both the House of Representatives and the

Senate, and was governor of the state of Wisconsin between 1901 and 1906. He was a fierce opponent of corporations and a lifelong crusader against government corruption, and he worked to reform government and get

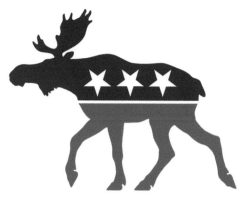

The Bull Moose Party was one of the most successful third parties in US political history.

progressive laws passed. La Follette also pushed for women's suffrage, racial equality, and fair representation of the populace. His opposition to corporate interests made him an outsider, even within the more liberal Republican Party.

In 1912, Roosevelt was selected over La Follette to represent the Progressive Party in the national election. As a member of what was popularly called the "Bull Moose Party," Roosevelt campaigned for progressive policies, such as universal suffrage, legislation to prevent industrial accidents, empowerment of labor unions, the abolition of child labor and convict-contract labor, and an overall stronger regulation of business. Though the Progressive Party performed well (better than any other third party in American history), it effectively split the vote with the Republican Party, allowing Democrat Woodrow Wilson to become president. After this defeat, the Progressive Party experienced a swift decline. Most progressives returned to the Republican Party, while some defected to the Democratic Party. La Follette later ran as a Progressive Party candidate for president in 1924, but he was only able to carry his home state.

## The Realignment of the Major Political Parties

Though the Progressive Party failed as a standalone political party, progressive ideas were nonetheless pursued by some representatives within the two major parties. While progressivism originally arose within the Republican Party, new social and economic programs increasingly came from Democratic politicians. For example, in response to the Great Depression, Democrat Franklin Delano Roosevelt began to adopt positions focused on workers' rights and social reforms. Roosevelt's so-called New Deal policies began to shift progressivism away from an exclusively Republican ideology.

After FDR's presidency, social change was the hot-button topic. With the economy finally booming again after the end of World War II, more people began to call for civil rights for all Americans. Politicians from both the Republican and Democratic Parties sought to implement sweeping reforms that ended "separate but equal" provisions in laws, which kept African Americans from attending schools alongside whites and permitted businesses to discriminate against African Americans.

It wasn't a single party that was responsible for pushing these reforms. Democratic politicians such as John F. Kennedy and Robert Kennedy pushed for drastic and complete civil rights reforms. Republican president Dwight Eisenhower supported desegregation and called in the National Guard to oversee the racial integration of Little Rock Central High School. At the same time, however, many people in both parties felt abandoned and betrayed by their political party due to these social reforms.

These progressive social policies were partially responsible for the realignment of the Republican and

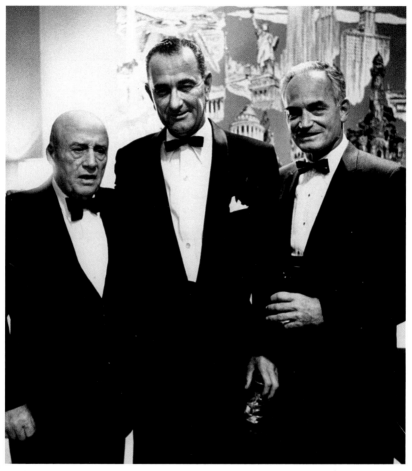

Lyndon B. Johnson (*center*) and Barry Goldwater (*right*) attend a dinner in 1959.

Democratic Parties. While the Democratic Party was once the conservative, anti-integration party of the South, it began taking on a new identity as a progressive party that sought social and economic reform. Meanwhile, the Republican Party began to appeal to conservative voters who saw some or all of these reforms as being bad for the country or as limiting individual freedoms. These new positions were solidified in 1964, when Barry Goldwater consolidated power in the Republican Party and received the party's presidential nomination. Goldwater was a staunch opponent of the Civil Rights Act of 1964. He lost the presidential election to incumbent Lyndon B. Johnson, but new political lines had been drawn. The Republican Party became the party of conservatives, and the Democratic Party became the liberal party. Most people who considered themselves to be progressives then left the Republican Party and either joined the Democratic Party or became independent voters.

## Progressive Social Policies Today

Today, progressives are gaining a stronger voice within the Democratic Party. In 2008, Barack Obama was elected president, and during his eight-year administration, he was able to pass several social reforms. He signed the Affordable Care Act, which provided health insurance to many underinsured and uninsured Americans. He signed the Dodd-Frank Act, which established stricter regulations on the financial sector and prevented firms from taking on certain risks. Most of Obama's reforms were opposed by conservative politicians who believed that the government already had too much influence over the health-care and financial industries. They saw such regulations as being anticompetitive and preferred to let the free market reward good business practices and punish bad ones. While Republicans did not wield the political power to block legislation during much of Obama's presidency, they did force concessions on some of the policies, restricting how far the government was allowed to legislate these industries.

With the election of President Donald Trump, many of these progressive reforms have been challenged, and some have been repealed. The Affordable Care Act has been targeted for repeal numerous times since Trump's election, and the Dodd-Frank Act has been modified to remove many

# Compromise in Government

Because people from a broad variety of ideologies believe that they know what's best for the country, it is very easy for them to become entrenched in their views and unwilling to listen to others. However, in order to achieve their goals, politicians often seek ways to compromise with those who have different perspectives.

When politicians want to write progressive laws, they often need to offer concessions on their ideology to make progress toward what they consider a greater good. One recent example of this came with the passage of the Affordable Care Act. In the face of growing health-care costs and millions of uninsured Americans, progressive politicians pitched the idea of a federally funded health-care system. Many conservative leaders and less-progressive members of Congress did not want the government to enter into the health insurance market, fearing that it would ruin competition in the marketplace and drive many insurance companies out of business. After much deliberation, one of the compromises that politicians reached was to allow the government to subsidize payments to private insurance companies for lower-income individuals but prevent the government from offering its own coverage to all people. By paying portions of the premiums for lower-income individuals, the government would expand health-care coverage for people who didn't have access to health care before the Affordable Care Act was passed.

While progressive politicians felt the need to back away from some of the more radical pieces of the law, they did succeed in achieving many of their goals. And while conservatives prevented the government from becoming an insurance provider, they had to compromise by allowing health insurance to be mandatory.

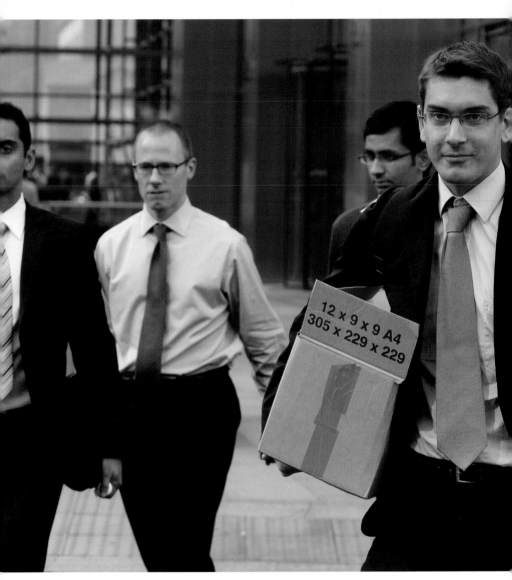

Men leave a Lehman Brothers office in London, England, on September 15, 2008, after the US investment bank's announcement that it would file for bankruptcy protection.

of the regulations that President Obama signed into law in 2010. While the Affordable Care Act remains in place for now, there have been many attempts to undercut its funding sources and to limit its impact. A decrease in financial regulation seems to have led to stock-market gains, but progressives warn that stripping key regulations may cause another financial collapse in the future.

The rollback of these reforms has energized progressives within the Democratic Party. Even as the Republican Party drifts rightward–conservatives are considered "right-wing" while liberals are "left-wing"–the Democratic Party is drifting leftward, away from the more moderate and compromising positions it has taken for the last few election cycles. More progressive candidates are winning their primaries against longtime Democratic incumbents. The mood of the country seems to be changing, as are the demographic and ideological makeup of the population.

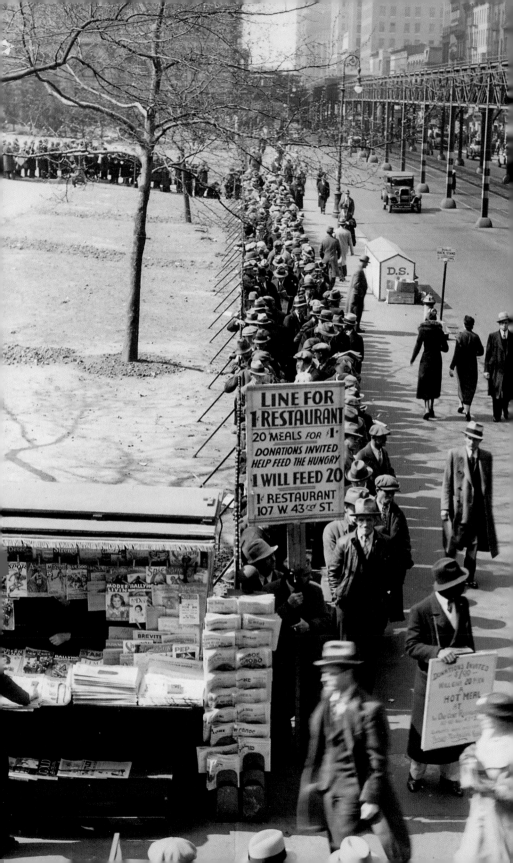

LINE FOR
1¢ RESTAURANT
20 MEALS FOR 1¢
DONATIONS INVITED
HELP FEED THE HUNGRY
I WILL FEED 20
1¢ RESTAURANT
107 W. 43rd ST.

# Chapter 3

# Progressivism and the Economy

While conservatives would prefer that the government stay out of economic matters, progressives feel that government intervention is necessary. They argue that unfettered capitalism is inherently exploitative of the middle and lower classes because it concentrates the wealth of a nation in the hands of relatively few people.

To help regulate and prevent this concentration of wealth, progressives favor government intervention in the form of taxes and restrictions on business. They also push to improve working conditions and enact strict consumer-protection laws. In an ideal progressive economy, workers would share in the profits of the business and have a safe and clean working environment. The country as a whole would work to preserve natural resources and ensure consumer protections, even if it means less profit for businesses.

## The Industrial Revolution

In the early 1900s, progressive policies became popular in response to the modernization of America. As factories

*Opposite*: People wait in a breadline in New York City at the height of the Great Depression, circa February 1932.

became more and more common, the poor working conditions within these factories became better known to the public. Labor unions and progressive government policies limited the free market by enacting many more restrictions, both on the consumer end and the production end. Progressive policies are usually pro-union because progressives see unions as a way to combat the power that wealthy business owners have in a capitalistic society.

Before the Industrial Revolution, the US government mostly stayed out of the marketplace. People were allowed to found their businesses and sell their products at whatever prices they wanted with little oversight. When factories became more common and production ramped up, trading within the American economy increasingly occurred on a national–rather than local–level. Soon, people were able to buy mass-produced goods from around the country at lower prices. Smaller farms started disappearing, skilled craftspeople were driven out of business, and people began flocking to cities in search of employment in the mills and factories. As production became concentrated into the hands of fewer companies, it became much easier to exploit people for labor. In response, workers began electing officials who promised to introduce some level of oversight to these factories.

## Poor Working Conditions

One of the key ways that progressives want the government to intervene in economic issues is through the regulation of working conditions so that they are more favorable to labor, even if they become less favorable to management in the process. In the late 1800s and early 1900s, large factories began replacing family farms as the primary way people earned a living. As people moved from the countryside into the cities, these new factories could draw from a large labor pool.

Because many positions in the factories were for unskilled labor, there was a huge supply of laborers for a limited number of jobs. Experienced workers could be easily replaced for any reason, so wages were kept low and the incentive to keep workers happy was nonexistent. After all, if someone got hurt or didn't feel as though they were paid enough, there were thousands of people who could replace him or her.

Conditions in these factories were often brutal. With no safety restrictions in place, people would get hurt while working, only to be fired because they could no longer perform the functions of their job. In the early 1900s, thousands of workers died every year in workplace

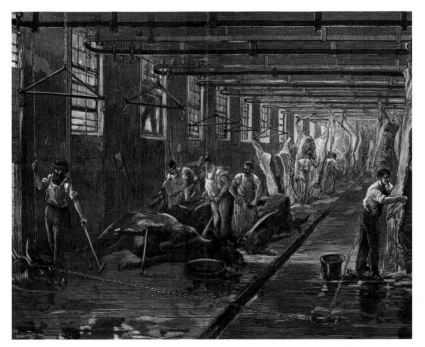

The meat-packing industry was one of the larger employers of immigrant labor in Chicago in the early 1900s.

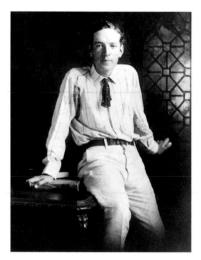

Upton Sinclair wrote books and articles to highlight the abuses suffered by American factory workers.

accidents and from illness due to unsanitary conditions. While these conditions were widespread among the whole population, they acutely affected immigrant populations. Because these new Americans were often poor, had few connections outside of their family and immediate communities, and had no political voice, these people were likely to be exploited. They also faced opposition from nonimmigrant laborers who believed they were oversaturating the work market and driving down wages.

Not only were adult men exploited as laborers, but women and children often worked in the factories as well, usually for much less money than was paid to men. Because of such low wages, entire families needed to work to support themselves. For many families, however, it was still nearly impossible to make enough money to save for emergencies, medical care, or retirement. One person getting injured on the job could drive the entire family to starvation.

Upton Sinclair was a writer and journalist who noticed how poorly people were being treated and became committed to exposing the conditions in which these people worked. In 1905, he published a novel depicting an immigrant family working in the stockyards of Chicago. While the family was fictionalized, the working conditions and food contamination that Sinclair described in *The Jungle* were very real, and the book convinced many Americans that change needed to happen. *The Jungle* caused such a stir that it helped pass the Pure Food and Drug Act and the Meat Inspection Act in 1906, which regulated what could be in food that was packaged and consumed by the American people. These progressive reforms, enacted at the federal level, met with resistance from those who believed that the free market was being unfairly hindered. With these initial successes, however, politicians began working together to push for even more economic reforms.

## Economic Responses to the Great Depression

In response to the Great Depression of the 1930s, President Franklin D. Roosevelt proposed a series of programs that he said would help kick-start the economy and get people back to work. This New Deal promised relief for the unemployed, economic recovery, and the reform of capitalism. It placed the responsibility of the citizens' well-being in the government rather than in individual companies, and provided assurance from the federal government that steps would be taken to change how the economy worked.

Within the first few months of becoming president, Roosevelt introduced legislation that manipulated the supply and price of agricultural products in an attempt to stabilize those markets. Conservatives do not like it when the government regulates how the economy functions by setting artificial prices or changing supply because they feel the market operates more efficiently on its own. Progressives, however, argued that it was necessary to intervene in this case because farmers did not have enough demand for their crops. After European farmers recovered from World War I,

American farmers were producing more food than could be consumed. Without the ability to sell their crops, farmers were not able to hire people to help harvest or plant them. The entire agricultural economy stagnated, so the government intervened to help stabilize the market.

Roosevelt also wanted to impose regulations on the banking and financial industries, which he saw as taking unnecessary risks and harming the American people in the process. By creating the Federal Deposit Insurance Corporation (FDIC), Roosevelt required that all banks become insured by the federal government. This meant that if the bank went out of business due to bad investments, the federal government would cover the losses of the people

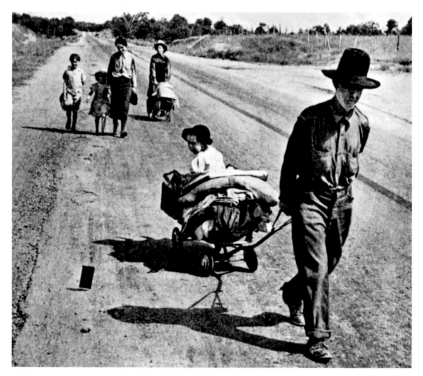

A Midwestern farmer and his family are forced to abandon their farm in 1930s America as crops fail and unemployment soars during the Great Depression.

who deposited their money in that bank. This encouraged confidence in banks and pushed more people to keep their money in them. Meanwhile, the Securities and Exchange Commission (SEC) introduced oversight and regulation to the stock market, which was partially to blame for the downward spiral of the economy. The SEC was empowered to investigate and punish bad actors to help keep the stock market more stable.

Roosevelt also guaranteed workers' right to organize into unions, while also establishing requirements for industry wages and prices. In the past, the government had helped to break up unions in order to help businesses increase their profits. So, by guaranteeing the right to organize, Roosevelt helped ensure that there would be a check on the power wielded by corporations. New laws also established federally mandated wages and industry-specific prices. This forced companies to pay workers a minimum wage and prevented labor surpluses from driving down wages. By setting prices, the government was able to better control spending and encourage economic activity among the population.

Not content to regulate existing industry, the New Deal also created new jobs working for the federal government. The Works Progress Administration (WPA) started employing people to build public infrastructure. Roads, bridges, public schools, hospitals, and sewer systems were constructed by government employees. These programs were meant to help decrease unemployment and give unskilled laborers a job that they could do while private industry adapted to the new economic environment. As defense production increased during World War II, these government employees were able

# The Planned Economy

Many people today use the terms "progressivism" and "socialism" interchangeably. While there are similarities between these two ideologies, there are also some key differences—one of which concerns the idea of a planned economy. In a socialist society, the government plays a role in dictating what businesses produce and how much they create. Critics of this system say that it stifles creativity and hinders economic growth. Proponents of a centrally planned economy believe that it prevents scarcity in key products and services, and that with careful planning, the economy can remain strong.

A progressive society favors government intervention but does not believe that the economy should be centrally planned. Instead, progressives want the government to regulate practices to prevent inequality and to promote safety, on behalf of both consumers and laborers. They also want to ensure that natural resources are protected for all citizens. In a progressive society, the government does not control the economy but instead guides the economy by penalizing bad behavior and offering incentives for good behavior. For example, progressives favor stronger environmental protections, even if it means that certain companies, such as coal and oil providers, will lose profits.

Many progressives also prefer companies to be cooperatively owned by the people who work there. This way, as the company succeeds, profits are shared by those who take part in the production of goods. Because progressives believe that capitalism is inherently exploitative of the working class, they feel that encouraging or requiring companies to be collectively owned helps prevent that exploitation. This also

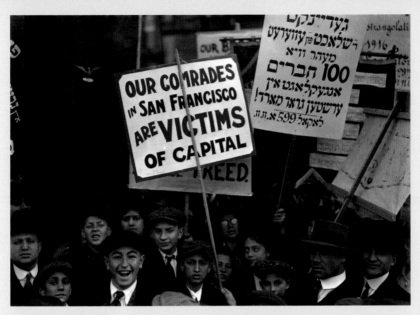

West Coast dock strikers critique capitalism in 1916. Striking is one way that workers can try to demand better working conditions and pay from their employers.

promotes more participation in the economy by more people, preventing the mass accumulation of wealth in the hands of a few business owners.

While progressives would like to see the entire economic system replaced with a more worker-centric model, most recognize that this will take time and effort from a lot of people. Therefore, the current, shorter-term goals are to help pass laws that strengthen unions, enact regulations that limit environmental impact, and pay for social services by taxing the wealthy people who profit most from the nation's economy.

to find work in the private sector, and the WPA was disbanded in 1943. Providing work for unemployed people during the Great Depression cemented government involvement in the American economy for decades to come.

## Progressive Economic Policies Today

Today, some of the progressive policies implemented during the first half of the twentieth century have come under fire. Labor unions in certain states face new legislation that limits their bargaining power, and unions have faced public pressure for perceived corruption. As of 2018, twenty-seven states had implemented "right to work" laws that restrict how unions can collect dues and whether an employee can be required to join the union associated with a particular company. These changing laws have diminished the effectiveness of unions in recent years. Progressives who support stronger unions believe that they are more relevant than ever, and that the government should return some of the bargaining power that labor unions enjoyed in the post–World War II years.

Meanwhile, some federal regulation agencies have had their power lessened in recent years. The Environmental Protection Agency, once charged with punishing bad actors by leveraging fines against corporations that do not follow environmental legislation, has become a more lenient, business-friendly agency. Former restrictions on greenhouse gas emissions have been rolled back, and incentives for clean energy have been reduced. Some say that these changes have a positive impact on the economy, but progressives argue that these rollbacks have led to negative environmental impacts.

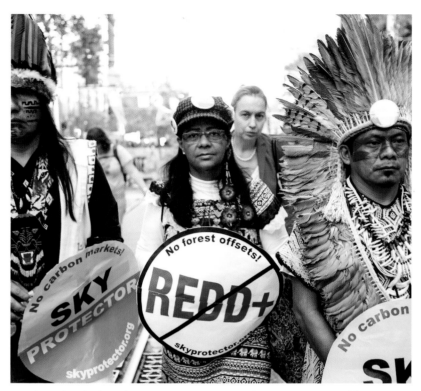

Members of a tribe from the Amazon Rain Forest march in San Francisco, California, on September 8, 2018, to demand meaningful solutions to climate change.

Newly enacted federal legislation has shifted from reflecting more progressive ideologies under the Obama administration to more conservative ideologies under the Trump administration. Where progressives want to support the lower, middle, and working classes by offering public services and economic protections, conservatives want to offer benefits to people who own and run businesses in the belief that free-market competition will not only help the middle and lower class but also expand American prosperity.

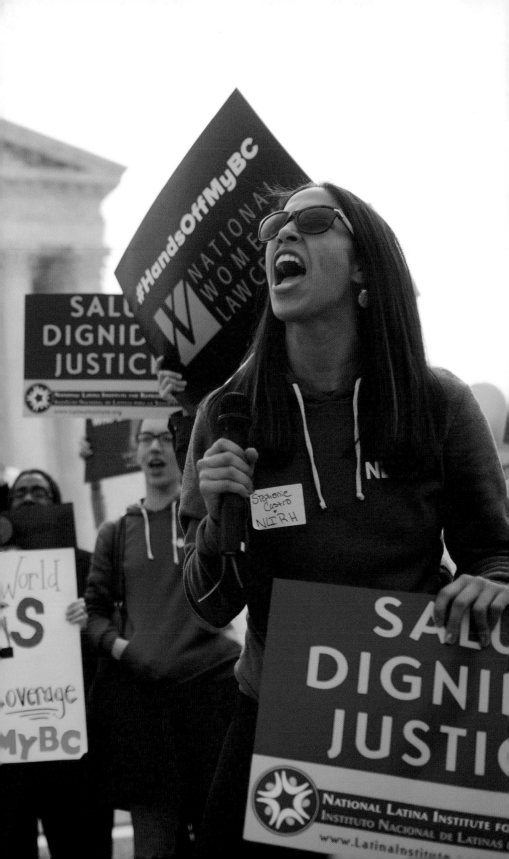

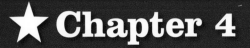

# ★ Chapter 4

## Progressivism and Society Today

Aﬁer the 2016 election, the Democratic Party had to examine why it sustained such losses at the state and national level. While there was disagreement as to why Democrats performed so poorly, one thing was certain—if the Democratic Party was to survive, it would have to adapt to the changing political climate. One of the factions leading the charge in changing the party is the progressive faction.

### Progressivism after the 2016 Election

Democratic candidates in recent elections were mostly centrist candidates who tried to appeal to moderate and independent voters. However, in the 2016 presidential election, Democratic senator Bernie Sanders ran a more progressive campaign than his fellow Democratic frontrunner, Hillary Clinton. When Sanders lost the Democratic Party nomination, many of his supporters were disheartened at the party itself and became more likely to either abstain from

*Opposite:* Pro-choice demonstrators stand before the US Supreme Court on March 23, 2016, while the court hears testimony from religious organizations who are disputing the Affordable Care Act's requirement that employer health-care plans cover birth control.

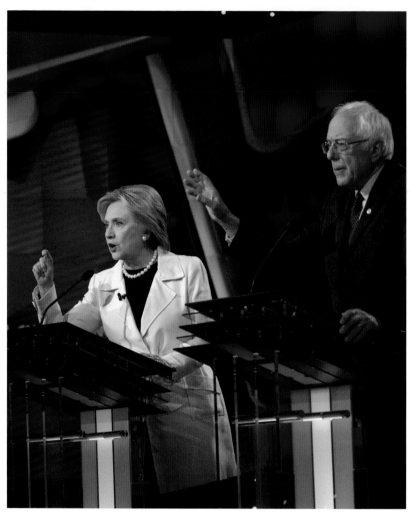

Presidential candidates Hillary Clinton and Bernie Sanders face off in a Democratic debate in 2016.

voting or to vote for third-party candidates such as Jill Stein of the Green Party. Stein, like Sanders, ran a campaign that appealed to more socialist and progressive voters.

It is likely Stein drew votes away from the more moderate Hillary Clinton, the Democratic presidential candidate. Much in the way that the Progressive Party split the election of

1912, support for these progressive candidates allowed for the Republicans to take control of the White House while maintaining their control of the Senate and the House of Representatives. While some people blame these third-party candidates and voters for causing Clinton to lose the election, others say that people should vote for whomever they want, and it's up to the candidate to appeal to the most voters.

When the moderate approach didn't work to win the presidency, the progressive wing started pushing for the Democratic Party to take a stance that was farther to the left. They believed that by becoming more extreme and vocal about the reforms they were looking to enact, they could harness the excitement and energy that was lacking in the previous election.

Longtime incumbents were challenged by new, more progressive candidates, sometimes forcing centrist candidates to start supporting more progressive policies. Some of these new candidates even won their primaries against the Democratic incumbents, receiving the nomination to run in the 2018 midterm elections. For example, in 2018, Alexandria Ocasio-Cortez challenged Joe Crowley, a longtime incumbent congressman, for the Democratic nomination in New York's Fourteenth Congressional District. Ocasio-Cortez ran on a platform that advocated many progressive policies, such as universal health care and a commitment to renewable energy for environmental reasons. She defeated Crowley in the primary and won a seat in the US House of Representatives in the 2018 midterm election.

Although other progressive Democrats were less successful in the 2018 midterms, some point to Ocasio-Cortez's successful primary bid as evidence that a truly progressive politician can win votes and be elected at the

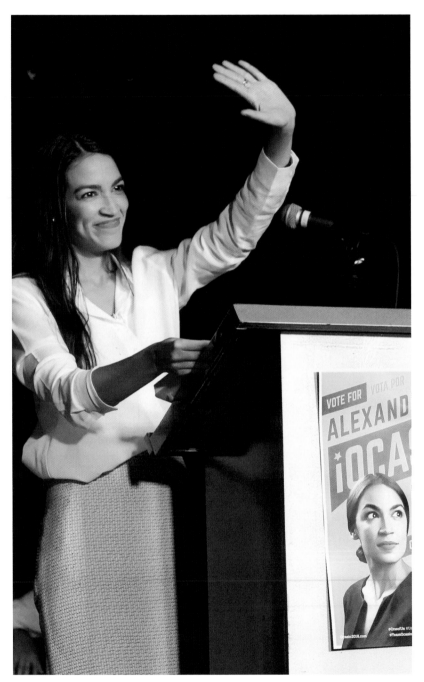

In the 2018 midterm elections, progressive candidates such as Alexandria Ocasio-Cortez, pictured here, won out against more moderate Democratic candidates in several districts.

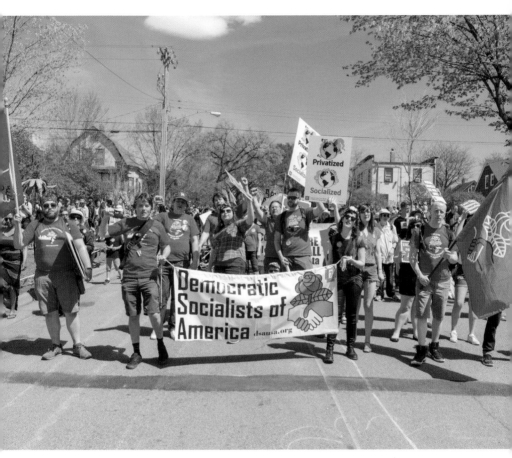

The Democratic Socialists of America is a group that works to elect progressive candidates.

national level. Much of the energy and excitement behind such campaigns is fueled by disapproval of President Trump and his rollback of progressive policies. Progressives believe that this energy can be harnessed and used to win more elections. If enough people who support progressive policies are elected, they will have the political bargaining power to enact their preferred reforms.

One of the main organizations lobbying for progressive reforms is the Democratic Socialists of America (DSA). This group is not a political party, but instead endorses candidates

# The Nordic Model

Many American progressives look to the Nordic model as representative of how progressivism could reshape a capitalistic society such as that of the United States. The Nordic model is the economic and social system that Norway, Sweden, Finland, Denmark, Iceland, and the Faroe Islands follow. The model has been successful in these countries, and progressives argue that it demonstrates that capitalism can exist without the massive disparities in personal wealth that occur in the American system.

At the foundation for the Nordic model is a social safety net that includes a strong welfare program, ongoing

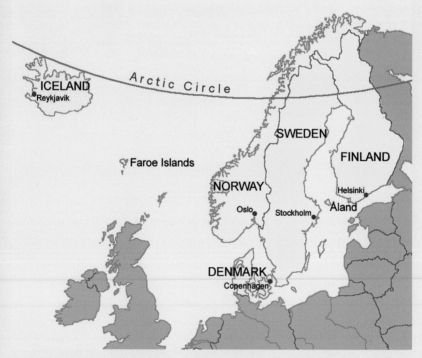

Many progressives see the Nordic model, inspired by the nations pictured here in yellow, as a framework for how to implement progressive policies in the United States.

unemployment benefits, a federally funded pension plan, and government-provided education and health care. These services are offered by the government and paid for with a high tax rate, both on corporations and on individuals. Proponents of this model argue that by offering all of these social benefits, the government encourages people to participate in their communities and prevents them from falling too far if they are unsuccessful. Opponents of the Nordic model believe that savvy business practices should be rewarded with money and economic success, and that when the government takes away such incentives, it diminishes people's drive to work hard.

Further, the Nordic model requires that strong labor unions bargain with corporate leaders to set wages, prices, and benefits. All of this is moderated by the government, which is there to ensure that people act in good faith and follow through on their agreements. Except for Norway, the countries that use the Nordic model are primarily home to privately owned companies that pay high taxes. Norway has several large, state-owned businesses, mostly involved in oil production, in addition to privately owned companies.

Many American progressives believe that by following the Nordic model and offering more protections and services to its citizens, the United States could stem the tide of inequality and avoid some of the worst aspects of capitalism, instead pursuing a kinder, more humane approach.

who support progressive policies and promise to pursue these policies if they are elected. The DSA operates on the federal and state level, and acts as an organizer for voters. Among its objectives are stronger union representation, higher taxes for the wealthy, and better public services. To be sponsored by the DSA, a politician needs to commit to certain progressive policy reforms, specifically strengthening unions and providing health care for all US citizens.

Most groups such as the DSA know that they will not succeed in changing the system overnight. Instead, they argue that progressivism is about working within a society to enact social and economic change. Progressives do not want a true revolution, but rather a deliberate movement toward a more equitable society.

## The Future of Progressivism

As a member of the global community, the United States affects and is affected by what other countries do and the policies they enact. While many European nations are more progressive than the United States, in recent years many of these progressive reforms have been falling out of favor. In 2016, a conservative campaign to get the United Kingdom to leave the European Union succeeded, backed primarily by people who believed that economic restrictions put in place by the EU were hindering the economy. This "Brexit," or "British Exit," continues to be a point of contention in European politics.

Other conservative candidates have won support in longtime progressive nations. Marine Le Pen took second in the 2017 presidential election in France after pushing for a more conservative and nationalist government. Such elections will help shape the world in the coming years.

Progressives continue to position themselves in opposition to a system that they see as heartless, cruel, and alienating. For evidence of the failure of current capitalist structures, progressives point to the disconnect between production and producer, especially in the global economy; to long working hours and stagnating wages; and to companies that are seeing record profits without distributing those profits to their employees in a way that progressives consider equitable. Progressives in the United States continue to push for legislation that reforms business practices, provides social aid to citizens, and protects the people whom they consider most vulnerable to persecution.

**1890** Sherman Antitrust Act is signed, regulating competition among companies.

**1905** Upton Sinclair publishes *The Jungle*.

**1906** Theodore Roosevelt signs the Pure Food and Drug Act, setting standards for what contents and contaminants can be included in food that is sold on the market.

**1906** Theodore Roosevelt establishes new national parks, preserves, forests, and other conservation programs dedicated to preserving natural resources. He also establishes the US Forest Service.

**1912** Theodore Roosevelt runs for president as a Progressive Party candidate, splitting the vote with William Howard Taft and paving the way for Democrat Woodrow Wilson to win the election.

**1929** The US stock market crashes, plunging the United States into the Great Depression.

**1933** Franklin Delano Roosevelt becomes president. Many cultural and economic reforms follow, including the Social Security Act and the Civilian Conservation Corps.

**1964** The Civil Rights Act outlaws racial segregation in schooling, employment, and both public and private services.

**1964** Barry Goldwater wins the Republican presidential nomination, redrawing political borders based on conservatism and liberalism rather than north/south boundaries.

**2007** A financial crisis in the banking industry causes several large banks and financial firms to collapse. Global economic downturn follows.

**2010** President Barack Obama signs the Affordable Care Act into law. Obama also signs the Dodd-Frank Wall Street Reform and Consumer Protection Act, establishing more rules and regulations for the financial sector.

**2016** Donald Trump is elected president. Conservatives start pushing for the repeal of progressive financial and health-care reforms.

**2019** Newly elected progressive Democrat Alexandria Ocasio-Cortez proposes the Green New Deal, a broad framework for fighting climate change inspired by the scope of the New Deal, Franklin Roosevelt's programs for recovering from the Great Depression.

# Glossary

**Affordable Care Act**  A law signed in 2010 that expanded health-care coverage to almost all Americans.

**capitalism**  An economic system where private owners control production for profit.

**compromise**  People of differing ideologies working together to create reforms.

**conservatism**  A political ideology that generally supports a weaker federal government and less government involvement in the economy.

**constituents**  People who are represented by a politician.

**Dodd-Frank Act**  A law passed in 2010 that placed stricter regulations on the financial industry with the goal of avoiding another financial crisis like the Great Recession of 2007-2009.

**empirical**  Originating in or based on evidence or observation.

**Enlightenment**  A philosophical movement emphasizing reason and individualism, and urging that more people should have a say in their government.

**ideology**  An overarching system of thought that shapes a person's beliefs and actions.

**incentive**  Something that promotes or incites a particular action.

**incumbent**  The candidate who already holds a political office and is running to keep it.

**individualism**  A doctrine that supports the interests of the individual above those of the group.

**Industrial Revolution**  A period of time when new manufacturing processes arose, moving away from hand-production to factories and machine tools.

**labor union**  A group of workers who band together to bargain for benefits and reforms.

**liberalism**  An ideology that generally favors higher taxes and a strong federal government in return for more social safety nets and government protections.

**mass production**  The manufacture of large quantities of standardized products, usually by assembly line.

**midterm election**  The election that occurs two years into a president's term.

**moderate**  Someone who holds both liberal and conservative opinions, who might vote for a Republican in one election and a Democrat in another.

**New Deal**  A set of programs enacted to bring relief to people suffering during the Great Depression.

**progressivism**  An ideology based on an empowered workforce and robust public services based on higher taxes.

**Pure Food and Drug Act**  A law signed in 1906 that establishes what foreign objects and substances can be in food, and in what quantities.

**republic**  A form of government in which citizens elect representatives to government and elect a president rather than a monarch.

**schism**  The splitting up of a group based on ideological differences.

**Securities and Exchange Commission**  A government office that enforces financial laws.

**"separate but equal"**  A legal doctrine that allowed segregation to exist in the United States without violating the Fourteenth Amendment.

**socialism**  A political theory that advocates for the means of production to be owned by the community as a whole.

**subsidize**  When the government pays for all or part of a good or service.

**suffrage**  The right to vote.

**third-party candidate**  A candidate who runs not as a Democrat or a Republican. Third-party candidates are often ideologically similar to one of the main candidates, and draw votes away from that person.

**unfettered**  Without restrictions.

**Works Progress Administration**  A program established by Franklin Roosevelt that employed people to build national infrastructure.

## Books

Cochran, Molly, and Cornelia Navari, eds. *Progressivism and US Foreign Policy Between the World Wars*. New York: Palgrave Macmillan, 2017.

Pearson, Sidney A., Jr. *Reflections on American Progressivism*. New Brunswick, NJ: Transaction Publishers, 2014.

Sicius, Francis J. *The Progressive Era: A Reference Guide*. Santa Barbara, CA: ABC-CLIO, LLC, 2015.

Wolraich, Michael. *Unreasonable Men: Theodore Roosevelt and the Republican Rebels Who Created Progressive Politics*. New York: Palgrave Macmillan, 2014.

Woolner, David B., and John M. Thompson, eds. *Progressivism in America: Past, Present, and Future*. New York: Oxford University Press, 2016.

## Websites

**National Women's History Museum: Progressive Era**

https://www.womenshistory.org/education-resources/topics/progressive-era

The National Women's History Museum offers a look at the social justice reforms targeted by important progressive women in the early twentieth century.

**The Progressive Era**

https://www2.gwu.edu/~erpapers/teachinger/glossary/progressive-era.cfm

This site contains a brief overview of the Progressive Era along with links to primary documents, other websites, and further information about the people of the era.

**Progressive Era Toolkit**
http://teachingamericanhistory.org/american-history-toolkits/
progressive-era-toolkit
This site offers primary documents on the Progressive Era,
along with some interesting questions to think about while
researching progressivism.

## Videos

**How Progressivism Happened**
https://www.youtube.com/watch?v=tfUYi8ehLMk
In this video, we see how the rise of the Progressive Party split
the Republican vote in the early twentieth century, allowing
Woodrow Wilson to win the presidency. The video also
explains how the progressive movement started.

**The Labor Movement in the United States**
https://www.youtube.com/watch?v=ewu-v36szlE
This video recalls some of the labor riots during the Industrial
Revolution and explains how labor unions pushed for
work reforms.

**The Progressive Era: Crash Course US History**
https://www.youtube.com/watch?v=i0Q4zPR4G7M
This video is an overview of the Progressive Era, focusing on
the social and economic changes spurred on by advances
in manufacturing.

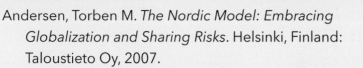

Andersen, Torben M. *The Nordic Model: Embracing Globalization and Sharing Risks*. Helsinki, Finland: Taloustieto Oy, 2007.

"Dodd-Frank Wall Street Reform and Consumer Protection Act: Conference Report (to Accompany H.R. 4173)." Washington, DC: US Government Publishing Office, 2010.

"Employer/Union Rights and Obligations." National Labor Relations Board. Accessed October 18, 2018. https://www.nlrb.gov/rights-we-protect/rights/employerunion-rights-and-obligations.

"Enlightenment." History.com. Accessed October 3, 2018. https://www.history.com/topics/british-history/enlightenment.

"FDA's Evolving Regulatory Powers, Part I: The 1906 Food and Drugs Act and Its Enforcement." US Food and Drug Administration. Accessed October 2, 2018. https://www.fda.gov/AboutFDA/History/FOrgsHistory/EvolvingPowers/ucm054819.htm.

Fisk, Donald M. "American Labor in the 20th Century." US Bureau of Labor Statistics, January 30, 2003. https://www.bls.gov/opub/mlr/cwc/american-labor-in-the-20th-century.pdf.

Flanagan, Maureen A. "Progressives and Progressivism in an Era of Reform." *Oxford Research Encyclopedia of American History*, August 2016. http://americanhistory.oxfordre.com/view/10.1093/acrefore/9780199329175.001.0001/acrefore-9780199329175-e-84.

"The Industrial Revolution in the United States." Library of Congress. Accessed October 18, 2018. http://www.loc.gov/teachers/classroommaterials/primarysourcesets/industrial-revolution.

Kelso, Randall R. "Styles of Constitutional Interpretation and the Four Main Approaches to Constitutional Interpretation in American Legal History." *Valparaiso University Law Review* 29 (1994).

"Labor Unions During the Great Depression and New Deal." Library of Congress. Accessed October 16, 2018. http://www.loc.gov/teachers/classroommaterials/presentationsandactivities/presentations/timeline/depwwii/unions.

"Minor/Third Party Platforms: Progressive Party Platform of 1912." American Presidency Project. Accessed October 18, 2018. http://www.presidency.ucsb.edu/ws/index.php?pid=29617.

"Party Affiliation." Gallup, 2018. https://news.gallup.com/poll/15370/party-affiliation.aspx.

Pear, Robert. "Negotiating to 60 Votes, Compromise by Compromise." *New York Times*, December 19, 2009. https://www.nytimes.com/2009/12/20/health/policy/20care.html.

Perlstein, Rick. "1964 Republican Convention: Revolution from the Right." *Smithsonian* magazine, August 2008. https://www.smithsonianmag.com/history/1964-republican-convention-revolution-from-the-right-915921.

"Robert M. La Follette." Biography.com, January 22, 2015. https://www.biography.com/people/robert-m-la-follette-40226.

Saad, Lydia. "U.S. Conservatives Outnumber Liberals by Narrowing Margin." Gallup, January 3, 2017. https://news.gallup.com/poll/201152/conservative-liberal-gap-continues-narrow-tuesday.aspx.

Stein, Jeff. "What Ocasio-Cortez Wants for America After Beating Joe Crowley." *Washington Post*, June 27, 2018. https://www.washingtonpost.com/news/wonk/wp/2018/06/27/ocasio-cortez-beat-joe-crowley-campaigning-on-medicare-for-all-guaranteed-jobs-and-abolishing-ice.

Strouse, Jean. *Morgan: American Financier*. New York: Random House, 2014.

"Upton Sinclair." Biography.com, May 22, 2017. https://www.biography.com/people/upton-sinclair-9484897.

"United States Presidential Election of 1912." *Encyclopædia Britannica*, October 4, 2016. https://www.britannica.com/event/United-States-presidential-election-of-1912.

Ward, J. S., G. L. Baker, and Wayne D. Rasmussen. *A Short History of Agricultural Adjustment, 1933–75*. United States Department of Agriculture, Economic Research Service, 1976.

"What Is Democratic Socialism?" Democratic Socialists of America (DSA). Accessed October 18, 2018. https://www.dsausa.org/about-us/what-is-democratic-socialism.

"What We Do." US Securities and Exchange Commission, June 10, 2013. https://www.sec.gov/Article/whatwedo.html#create.

"Wide Gender Gap, Growing Educational Divide in Voters' Party Identification." Pew Research Center, March 20, 2018. http://www.people-press.org/2018/03/20/1-trends-in-party-affiliation-among-demographic-groups.

"Works Progress Administration (WPA)." History.com. Accessed October 18, 2018. https://www.history.com/topics/great-depression/works-progress-administration.

# Index

Page numbers in **boldface** refer to images.

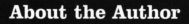

# About the Author

**Matt Bougie** is a writer and marketer from Friendship, Wisconsin, who currently lives in Milwaukee, Wisconsin. He is the author of several books, including *Strategic Inventions of the Cold War* and *The Bell Witch: Ghost of Tennessee.* Bougie enjoys reading and writing, especially about history and technology.

Young Adult
320.513
Bon